More

"*Tough Broad* is an entertaining read. It's sure to inspire women to continue to enjoy the outdoors, create new neural pathways as they try new things, and enjoy the camaraderie of their sisters in adventure into their later years."

—*USA Today*, "Outdoors Wire"

"This arc of a critical life blueprint comes from the toughest broad I know, Caroline Paul. You turn the last page of *Tough Broad* and promise yourself to spend every minute possible in the great outdoors. You are determined to test new horizons, to abandon your fears, to breathe your deepest breath. I'm seventy-four. Caroline leads those of us of mature and wise ages to the very real hope that we all of us have much more to explore."

—**Diana Nyad, the first person to swim from Cuba to Florida without a shark cage, at age sixty-four**

"In this inspiring book, Paul encourages women to embrace the exhilaration and vitality that come with an adventurous life."

—**AARP.org**

"Paul's storytelling here goes deep, exploring the nuances of each woman's quest to understand her own pull to outdoor adventure. *Tough Broad*, she writes, 'is not about bravado, it is about bravery.' And it is as engrossing as it is inspiring."

—*BookPage*

"Paul makes a strong case for how a positive attitude about getting older can lead to a longer, healthier life . . . Paul, who was one of the first women firefighters in San Francisco, encourages other women to stay active and intrepid in their postmenopausal life, profiling older women who surf, hike, scuba dive, and explore. She recommends taking empowering walks in astonishing places like the Grand Canyon and Niagara Falls. Women don't have to give in to age's changes; there's a big world out there to engage with and gain strength and pleasure from. Here's to being old, 'game,' and down for adventure."

—*Booklist*

"Growing old is not an excuse for eschewing adventure; on the contrary, Paul argues in this bracing book, hiking, camping, scuba diving, and a host of other activities are necessary for aging women to lead richer lives. Weaving her high-octane anecdotes together with research on septuagenarian—and even older—women, Paul invites women everywhere to forge a life full of excitement."

—*Alta* magazine

"New adventures help bring this book full circle in a wonderful way. Readers will be charmed and inspired to try something new, to move and dive and breathe, no matter what their age."

—*The Bookworm Sez*

"Paul emphasizes how we can embrace the changes that come in our life with daring courage and heartening spirit that are not just attributes of our youthful days. This book is for everyone. Young and old alike, it's a reminder to embrace lifelong learning, to face our fears with bravery, to challenge oneself to see with a new lens and overturn our culture's beliefs about age. There is a world of awe and wonder just waiting to be discovered, and there are sides to us that will otherwise lie dormant unless we take a step towards the growth found within adventure."

—*Explore* **magazine**

"Paul's excellent writing offered me instant connections, showing me a range of women who were adventuring at their own level and facing challenges in very relatable ways . . . *Tough Broad* is not just a series of examples of inspiring, adventurous broads. Paul weaves key elements of research on aging into each section, making herself and the various adventurers' examples of the research results in action . . . Let me say that if you think you want to shake up your activities a bit and try something new, Caroline Paul's *Tough Broad* is an excellent place to start . . . Paul's book has me fired up to find ways to get outdoors to have even more fun even more often and, as she recommends, to do it completely on my own terms."

—*Fit Is a Feminist Issue*

"Just as Paul's previous book appealed to older women, *Tough Broad*, though meant for older women, will likely inspire women decades younger . . . At eighty-four, Paul's mother told her daughter wistfully, 'What I would give to be sixty again. Do it now, before you can't.' That's good advice for any woman, or man, at any age."

—*The Hippo*

"Oh, how I love—and *need*—this book! Paul's subjects don't deny or mask their years: they embrace who they are with gusto and vitality, seizing the opportunity to enjoy, to grow, to challenge themselves mentally and physically. And they remind us of a fundamental truth about women and aging: Even as we become invisible to the culture, we become more visible—in the best of ways—to ourselves. I am *here* for you, tough broads!"

—**Peggy Orenstein,** *New York Times* **bestselling author of** *Unraveling*

"In *Tough Broad*, Caroline Paul takes the prevailing view of how women age—the 'long slow rot theory' of aging—and completely upends it. By masterfully pairing the latest research on aging along with stories of amazing, adventurous women who are taking risks and playing outdoors well into their eighties and beyond, she demonstrates that women can not only survive but thrive during this period of their lives. Prepare to be inspired!"

—**Juliet Starrett,** *New York Times* **bestselling author of** *Built to Move*, **and three-time Whitewater World Champion**

"Caroline Paul and her fellow tough broads know how to live life to the fullest. Every story in this book reminds us that life is truly what we make it and that our curiosity, love of the outdoors, and appetites for adventure don't have to end in middle or even old age."

—**Natalie Baszile, bestselling author of** *Queen Sugar* **and** *We Are Each Other's Harvest*

Tough Broad

The Gutsy Girl: Escapades for Your Life of Epic Adventure

Lost Cat: A True Story of Love, Desperation,
and GPS Technology (illustrated by Wendy MacNaughton)

Fighting Fire: A Memoir

East Wind, Rain: A Novel

Tough Broad

*From Bird-Watching to BASE Jumping—How
Outdoor Adventure Improves Our Lives as We Age*

Caroline Paul

BLOOMSBURY PUBLISHING
NEW YORK · LONDON · OXFORD · NEW DELHI · SYDNEY

BLOOMSBURY PUBLISHING
Bloomsbury Publishing Inc.
1359 Broadway, New York, NY 10018, USA
50 Bedford Square, London, WC1B 3DP, UK
Bloomsbury Publishing Ireland Limited,
29 Earlsfort Terrace, Dublin 2, D02 AY28, Ireland

BLOOMSBURY, BLOOMSBURY PUBLISHING, and the Diana logo
are trademarks of Bloomsbury Publishing Plc

First published in the United States 2024
This paperback edition published 2025

ISBN: HB: 978-1-63557-649-8; PB: 978-1-63973-636-2;
EBOOK: 978-1-63557-650-4

LIBRARY OF CONGRESS CATALOGING-IN-PUBLICATION DATA IS AVAILABLE

2 4 6 8 10 9 7 5 3 1

Typeset by Westchester Publishing Services
Printed in the United States by Lakeside Book Company, Harrisonburg, VA

To find out more about our authors and books visit
www.bloomsbury.com and sign up for our newsletters.

Bloomsbury books may be purchased for business or promotional use. For
information on bulk purchases please contact Macmillan Corporate and
Premium Sales Department at specialmarkets@macmillan.com.

For product safety–related questions contact productsafety@bloomsbury.com.

To Alexandra,
Beside me since the very beginning.
Twin, confidante, moral compass, first reader, tough broad.
Thank you, Black Jack.

CONTENTS

Tough Broad

SPIRIT

I

(Don't) Act Your Age

At every phase of your life, look at your options.
Please, don't pick the boring ones.

—BARBARA HILLARY, RETIRED NURSE, WHO SKIED TO
THE NORTH POLE AT SEVENTY-FIVE YEARS OLD

I approach the tollbooth at Yosemite National Park, already
wide-eyed at how the landscape has swelled from scuffed
flatlands into granite plinths, how telephone poles and stop
signs, inert, sentinel, have given way to the sway and glitter
of aspens. Even the clouds have shed their timidity, growing
biceps and triceps, flexing against the blue sky. No wonder
I'm impatient to leave the small box that is my automobile
and meet the wildness outside. In my mind's eye, I am already
catapulting myself across an alpine meadow like a young and

skittering seedling. I am already peering into the Merced River like so many snuffling elk before me.

Luckily, the line to enter the park is not long; it's well into autumn and the summer rush is over. Those who are here have persevered despite the haze of the worst wildfire season California has ever seen still bruising the air and the coronavirus just now receding from its second surge.

I roll down my window, and a young ranger leans from the tollbooth and politely asks for my ID and reservation paperwork—"paperwork" being a quaint description, since I hold up a phone instead—and all seems well, but then the young ranger says something else, which I don't catch, the masks we wear and the car noise around us making it hard to hear. I shake my head and cup my ear in the universal language of "What?" and she mimes an un-pinching of her thumb and forefinger and I understand that she is asking for the screen enlargement of the reservation name.

The name does not match my ID. Instead, it belongs to the friend who is entering at another gate, an hour from here. I explain that she booked the reservation for us; the plan is to meet inside the park.

"Your friend has to be present," the young ranger says, not unkindly. Her voice is resigned, making it clear that I am not the first numbskull to forget to adjust her bifocals (which I don't wear) to capture the fine print. "Sorry, but without her here, I can't let you bring your car in," she says.

I look for a sign that the ranger will relent, but she is young and earnest and rules are rules. For a moment there is an awkward silence that she fills with an apologetic cant of her head and a smoothing of her slightly shiny, chemically blended ranger shirt. "Do people walk?" I ask, and she looks alarmed and tells me it's nine miles to the valley. Then I remember my Onewheel, fully charged to its fifteen-mile capacity and resting in the trunk, so I say, half joking and half desperate, "Well, can I get on my Onewheel?"

I can see by her face that she doesn't understand so I add, "It's an electric skateboard," and she blinks rapidly, taking in the staid hatchback with the sensible gas mileage, the gray roots of my hair, the thin veil of cat dander that may be rising from my shirt, and the 1963 birth date on the ID. She repeats, "Electric skateboard?" as if giving me time to tell her I'm not serious, but I just nod and she pulls her head back in the booth, then reappears moments later and says that, um, sure, an electric skateboard is allowed.

"Okay, I'll be back," I say, and I watch her go momentarily still, as if already lost in the future of what she will compose on her social media feed—*Lolz! Old Lady, on skateboard!!!??* I don't hold this against her; when I was her age I was exactly the same, dumping everyone over fifty unceremoniously into a box labeled "Old," subdividing that further into just a few categories limited to adjectives like "Frail," "Ill," "Senile," or "Boring." Not to mention the big one: "Dying." From my callow, know-it-all perspective, everyone over fifty was on the downhill slide to imminent death. There was definitely no file labeled "Can Ride an Electric Skateboard." So, I don't feel resentful. I feel delighted and even a little bit sorry for my young ranger, who doesn't realize that soon enough she will be where I am. Then she will upend her own expectations (I hope), maybe even remembering this encounter thirty years on.

For now, though, she is still certain that the world works in a particular way, and that this is some sort of misunderstanding. She pins the politeness back on her face and waves me around in a U-turn. I park my car a quarter mile down the mountain. I put on my wrist guards and my helmet and my fanny pack (because I may be a skateboarder, but I am still fifty-seven years old and believe in safety first and quick access to ChapStick). I remove the Onewheel from the trunk, switch it on, then step back, admiring it. It's a balance board centered on one large wheel. Its rim is encircled with lights and a faint hum, all to indicate that the battery works and the gyroscopic innards are turning. It is, as I will soon explain to the rangers, a Segway married to a snowboard, but for all intents and purposes it is a just another branch from the family tree atop which sits the mighty skateboard. So that is how I explain it: an electric-powered skateboard-like thingamajig, shortened to "electric skateboard."

I put one foot on the rear side of the wheel and the other foot in front of it, push the board level, and suddenly I'm off, whizzing back up the winding road. I have a grin on my face, because how could I not? I'm outside. The air is crisp. All the marginalia I did not see the first time around from my sitting position in my car unfurls around me—the Merced River heaves and roils, granite rocks as big as hippos stampede along the banks, trees flash yellow and orange. Momentarily, magically, it feels as if I am connected back through time to all those humans before me who have gazed upon this landscape and caught their breath, amazed.

I approach the gate again and skirt the cars. Ahead lie those nine miles of windy mountain road: hacked and dynamited by the exhausted hands of laborers nearly a hundred years ago, then trod by horse, by stagecoach, by millions of automobiles and buses, yet surely territory rarely touched by skateboarders, certainly not by fifty-seven-year-old ladies on Onewheels. I zip toward a knot of rangers outside the hut, and as they turn toward me one shoots up her eyebrows as if she has spotted a black bear pawing, say, a lunch cooler—could be dangerous, don't do anything sudden, stay calm, the look says. Someone else laughs a little and they all stutter-step away from me as if I'm about to wipe out their entire squadron of youthful shins, but I stop and dismount without incident.

I've been riding my Onewheel since I was fifty-two, and it's often like this: From a distance, and in my helmet and sunglasses (and now my Covid mask) I look like any teenager hurtling forward with fearsome abandon. But as I approach and surge into closer focus, it becomes clear: I am your grandmother. Teenagers smirk and millennials grow wide-eyed, their thoughts as obvious as if enshrined in a talk bubble over their full heads of hair and jowl-less chins: Wait, what? That's an OLD WOMAN.

Come on, now, I'm not old. But at this moment, at the Yosemite gate, I am also not, by most cultural definitions, acting my age, and certainly not acting my gender; there might not be quite this kerfuffle if I were, say, an almost-sixty-year-old man. Yet who ruled that I shouldn't be on a skateboard? Who decreed that this type of fun was over for me?

I don't want to actually *be* younger. I love my late fifties, finding in them a solidity of self, a peace of mind, a true happiness unbuffeted by the insecurities and tumult of earlier years— youth's abject self-consciousness, hapless communication skills, and angst about everything ranging from appearance to sex to what everyone else is thinking. And yet, while riding the skateboard I do feel many things *attributed* to younger generations: physically vital, confident, carefree, even a little bit reckless. Youth has claimed these emotions as their own, fully expectant that I am too fragile and perhaps incompetent (not to mention incontinent) to pursue them, and certain that I no longer desire them at all. But they are wrong. I have been energized all my life by physical vitality, confidence, freedom, and risk. Why would I give them up now?

. . .

A few years ago, I wrote a book for middle-grade girls about the wonders of outdoor adventure and the importance of bravery for their confidence and fulfillment. Parents agreed— courage was essential for their daughters and the outdoors was a perfect teacher—and *The Gutsy Girl: Escapades for Your Life of Epic Adventure* quickly became a *New York Times* bestseller. Turns out, it wasn't just girls who read the book. Grown women were also drawn to it, often at a moment in their life when they needed bravery. Some read it post-divorce, others while recovering from illness, still others as they embarked on their first solo vacation. These readers ran the gamut in age, but many were over fifty. They emailed, or raised their hands at events, and told me that, while growing up, they hadn't been encouraged to get outside. "Is it too late for me?" they asked. "No," I told them, with the fervor of an evangelist. "It's never too late!"

I answered with a lot of enthusiasm but, frankly, not much evidence. Now, as my own horizon begins to glow with the number sixty, I look around to see many men my age along- side me paddling a surfboard or riding a skateboard or flying an experimental plane, but very few female peers. Isn't being outside a vital elixir? Isn't adventure enlivening, and an important challenge? Why, then, aren't older women out here with me? At some age—it probably lies within a range—many women start believing that they can't, or shouldn't, be out there. Out there, as in the out-of-doors. Out there, as in a little bit unruly, a little off the beaten path. Out there, as in learning something new (my friend John took up flying ultralights in his mid-sixties), out there as in pushing physical comfort zones (Andy, at seventy-two, still paddles his surfboard into frigid and heavy winter swells). I'm not speaking about freaky, hair-raising danger, or overwhelming physical stress. I'm talking about a version of outdoor adventure that fits the realities of our age but doesn't succumb to the falsehoods—that as older women we are fragile, possibly mentally dotty, certainly not qualified to do anything but take constant precautions. Let's face it, our biggest danger may not be a mountain bike, or a surfboard, or saying yes to a tandem skydive. Instead, the real peril for us as we age is a sedentary life that lacks pizzazz and challenge. And I'm a lifelong adventurer: surely, I can continue to defy societal messaging while also gracefully accepting the very real fact that my body *is* changing, that I *am* weaker, slower, creakier. Ultimately, I'm my best self in the outdoors—curious, brave, and present. That in turn gives me confidence and optimism. All these seem like character traits I should hold on to as I age.

Yet years after I had so blithely responded, "It's never too late to get outside," I see that most women think that it is, in fact, too late. Not true, I say to myself. And this time I will prove it. And so begins my quest to more fully explore the benefits of outdoor adventure for me and for my peers.

. . .

What is adventure, anyway? You're on an adventure when you're reaching for a goal you've set, feeling physically and mentally engaged, maybe learning something new. It's when you're pushing your comfort zone, and experiencing exhilaration. And having fun. Always fun. Adventure, I believe, is within the reach of almost everyone, in spite of the differences in our physical, fiscal, and social situations.

As you read this, are you already shaking your head? Perhaps you are in less than robust health and long ago decided that outdoor adventure is a pipe dream. Or there may be financial constraints—don't the sports commonly associated with the genre require prohibitively expensive equipment? Some might have very limited access; if rollick and novelty is to happen it has to do so directly outside the front door, in the surrounding neighborhood, where there may be no nearby parks to put the "outdoor" in outdoor adventure. Finally, many still face a long, grueling workday even as the seventies, even eighties, loom. Outdoor adventure may feel like a leisure activity only for the comfortably retired, and not something vital for well-being, on par, say, with the pharmaceuticals that are prescribed with some abandon and that many dutifully swallow every day.

All of these concerns are valid. Outdoor adventure has long been an exclusive activity, narrowly defined, for so many years seemingly open only to white people, and furthermore white, *wealthy* people. I want to be clear at the outset that this book is relevant for all women growing older, not just for those who are white, rich, and robust.

. . .

Before the pandemic, in my mid-fifties, I was living a life of adrenaline. I was an intrepid if clumsy surfer. I regularly paddled my stand-up paddleboard in the bay. I flew a motorized hang glider. I took my Onewheel on trails and roads. I sometimes skied in the backcountry. I snowshoed. If there was no other exercise option in sight, I would embrace without much thought an open-water swim, something my twin sister, Alexandra, also did regularly. (She is one of those superhuman types who signs up for eleven-mile open-water races and is inevitably one of just a few—of any gender or age—who finish. We are both dogged, and she is even more dogged than I.)

But I noticed changes. The obvious ones were physical. My body was stiff, and I was flummoxed by its softness. I was dismayed too by my face, which was sagging in all the expected ways. Like many people, I would look in the mirror and not really recognize myself. Inside, it is said, we all have an age, and mine was somewhere between thirty-seven and forty-two. I couldn't square the strange commas around my mouth and the looseness of my neck with that internal person. But I was also curious. Who was I becoming in this later stage of life?

I wanted to welcome aging, not fight it. Fighting it would be a waste of time, and I calculated, as many do at this stage, the years of physical and cognitive health that I might have left if I was lucky (twenty-five?), and if I wasn't (perhaps seven?)—a terribly inexact math, yes, but the numbers aren't the point. I simply needed to make the most of what I had left. To do that I would have to figure out: What parts of my old identity fit this new phase of my life? What aspects were simply vestigial habits from previous decades? Ultimately my goal was to look past the prevailing narratives and expectations about women's aging to find out: Can't we embrace this long, last phase of our life with excitement, wringing what is possible out of it, despite difficulties?

I believe that we can, and that one key may lie in a renewed relationship with outdoor adventure. In the ensuing pages, you will find an exploration, a quest, really, in the Arthurian tradition, to answer this, as I encounter women adventurers along the way who have a lot to teach me. They aren't Olympians. They aren't famous. They aren't even necessarily good at what they do. But each and every one of them offers lessons on how to optimize this next and last stage, with its changing cultural currency, brain challenges, physical diminutions, and evolving social-emotional needs.

Let's be clear: This is not a book about adrenaline, it is a book about exhilaration. It is not about bravado, it is about bravery. It is not about athleticism, it is about health. It is not about exclusivity, it is about inclusion. Finally, it is about fulfillment—a paean not just to outdoor adventure, but to *your* outdoor adventure.

. . .

Back at the Yosemite tollbooth, the assessment of who I am and what I'm capable of seems to have shifted with my arrival on my electric skateboard. As I accept a map that has been proffered and answer a few wide-eyed questions about the Onewheel, I can tell I have upended expectations. Yet the young rangers have also deemed me harmless. I'm a onetime zoological curiosity of sorts, a far outlier on an otherwise neatly plotted bell curve.

But here's what I haven't told them.

The friend whose name is on my reservation, who I am meeting, is also in her fifties. And she would also give them pause. But much, much more pause. She is a BASE jumper, someone who habitually dons a parachute, then hucks herself from *b*uildings, *a*ntennae, *s*pans, and *e*arth (thus the B-A-S-E of BASE jumpers). Tomorrow at dawn it will be earth, specifically the earth on the rim of Yosemite's fabled wall, El Capitan. This is, of course, illegal; there is even a Yosemite park jail for those caught doing it and, too, for those like myself who serve as accessories to their crimes. But right now, to the earnest, milling rangers, I am the antithesis of a future felon. I am an older white woman with a cockamamie hobby, and it is confirmed again that the reservation is needed for the car, not the human, and that I am free to continue on my, um, skateboard. I am sent off with genuine smiles and small shakes of the head. Then the young rangers turn back to their duties, naturally assuming that there will be no more surprises, that I am otherwise just another gal with a bird list and a picnic, meeting a friend for a gawp around the valley. If they hear from me again, they are sure, it will be because my friend stopped her large sedan in the middle of the road and traffic piled up behind us: that's the kind of ridiculous thing those older women do when they spot something flying in the wild, the young rangers have been told. They have no inkling that what might be flying in the wild is actually one of these older women. With no more thought, they wave the next car through.

Look for Inspiration

You're only courageous if you do something you are afraid of doing.

—Dervla Murphy, travel author,
solo bicyclist into her eighties

I'm serpentining down the steep Yosemite park road on my electric skateboard. The mobile reception is iffy, but I've managed to send a text that explains the situation. *At entry gate/reservation snafu/on a Onewheel.* Four miles in I receive an answer: Shawn Brokemond is on her way. *Look for van.*

Shawn is someone who, the first time I met her, basically told me to go jump off a bridge. Normally, that might insult me. Coming from Shawn, though, this was the highest of compliments. Shawn was psyched for me to jump off a bridge, or anything, for that matter, because as a BASE jumper she regularly hurls herself off high places, counts the required number of seconds while free-falling, opens a parachute, then floats to the ground.

BASE jumpers are a peculiar brand of adventurer. Think skydiving, but without the plane. This might make BASE jumping sound tamer to you, but you'd be mistaken. BASE jumpers jettison themselves from earthbound objects, facing the constant danger of an inadvertent smack into something solid as they hurtle past. While skydivers can drop themselves from planes at ten thousand feet or more, BASE jumpers are lucky to find a launch that tops a thousand, offering much less time to pull their chute. The sports seem different on an emotional level, too; skydivers want to feel close to heaven and part of the sky, while BASE jumpers seem to relish their heart-pounding proximity to earth.

I have long been intrigued with BASE jumping. Still, is intrigue enough to justify learning one of the most dangerous sports in the world? According to my wife, my mom, and many of my friends, the answer is a resounding no. Still, BASE jumping had hovered on my periphery for years, gaining traction as an outdoor sport just as I was finding my own way into the sky. I became instead a paraglider, which also necessitated stepping off a cliff, but eschewed the gut-wrenching free fall and the liminal moment of uncertainty between when the chute is pulled and when (if) it opens. Instead, paragliders dangle from huge, stable canopies inflated while still land-bound that look pleasingly like an airplane wing. But BASE jumping always held a bigger element of cool; it epitomized courage and confidence and exhilaration. This is why, when a mutual friend mentioned Shawn, I jumped at the chance to meet her. And I had another reaction—an undeniable surge of righteous pride. This was undeserved, of course. It wasn't me who was BASE jumping, after all. But still, I felt somehow vindicated. *Look!* I wanted to shout out loud. *Women over fifty can be badass!*

Many may be baffled as to why a fifty-two-year-old would want to taunt death or serious injury. Isn't that reserved for callow youth? Shawn hasn't yet explained her own reasons to me, but she has assured me it wouldn't take much to find out for myself. Maybe I could accompany her to the Perrine Bridge, a popular spot (and one of the few legal places to jump in the United States)? "You have experience with parachutes," she'd said on that first meeting. "It'll be no problem." As she described how I would ball the chute in one hand, jump, and merely fling it free to open—no complicated release handles, no exact timing necessary—I briefly imagined myself there with her, even though the thought made my stomach drop as we spoke.

Shawn told me about jumping from free-standing antennae, which are often so high it can take her an hour and a half to ascend the ladder to the tiny platform on top. She also jumps from electrical towers. "You climb them," she said, "and you're getting shocked and—"

"Shocked!?" I interrupted. "Shocked, as in . . . what?"

She explained that as you near the very top of the tower, you get hit by electrical currents. "Like static electricity, but times ten." She didn't seem to think this was a big deal. She told me that this actually made it easier to jump. "Because I'm a little afraid of heights," she added, shrugging as if to say, *See? That shock thing works out so well.*

"Hold it, what?" I yelped. "You're afraid of heights?"

Shawn takes contradictions in stride. Electric shocks, good! Heights, scary! Jumping off high things, *excellent*. But then again, she is a fifty-two-year-old African American woman who BASE jumps. She's also a grandmother. An ex–kindergarten teacher. A woman with a boy's name. And someone who describes herself as having once been afraid of most everything in the wilderness. Contradictions, complications, obstacles, difficulties? Not a problem. Thus, when Shawn told me I could BASE jump, I believed her. It wasn't a matter of *if she can do it, I can, too.* No, Shawn is clearly a superior being, of the superhero variety. She *looks* like a superhero, lithe and tall, finely muscled, with a steady gaze and shoulders perfectly shaped for a quiver of golden arrows. And she has a unique superpower: she not only flies, but persuades you to momentarily dream that you can fly, too.

Now I pull over to the side of the road, read Shawn's new text, and respond: *Look for the dork in the helmet and the brown checkered shirt.* Then I remount my ride. After a few more miles, I see the van. I raise my arms, headlights flash in response, and the van pulls over.

Shawn and I don't know each other that well. We've met in person just twice; to her I'm the goofy writer with some decent experience in the outdoors, who seems to be curious about aging and perhaps BASE jumping. But if Shawn had any hesitation about allowing me to accompany her on this (illegal) excursion, it is now gone with the sight of the Onewheel. She laughs and I laugh, which at this moment is the communication equivalent of *You are my people, I get you.* I throw the skateboard into the back seat next to what is clearly her parachute rig, and we head to the valley to meet up with the rest of the team and to begin our scout of El Capitan: the launch spot, the landing spot, the escape routes.

Tumbling from the van, I say hello to Bruce, Shawn's husband, and their friend and fellow BASE jumper Jimmy. Jimmy has been described to me as a human cannonball—no, really, Shawn explained earlier, he was shot out of cannons for the Ringling Brothers circus. There is still something about Jimmy that is cannonball-ish: not just a muscular solidity, but a feeling of constant forward momentum—laughing, telling jokes, hopping from foot to foot. He is a stolid reminder of the expedition's raison d'être—that this is freewheeling and fun, an adventure as much about camaraderie and kinetic joy as actual adrenaline. Bruce is almost his opposite: quiet, serious, fit in the way of a man who has discipline as well as good genes. He has years of BASE experience, too, and rounds out the team as the informal logician, the guy with an eye on the gear, who remembers not just the all-important parachute rigs but also, say, the food from the long drive down that has been left under the car seat, and who deftly removes it before it spoils or the bears find it.

. . .

El Capitan's famous granite face was formed by igneous rock, then shaved by glaciers and smoothed by wind and rain, and now remains under such geologic pressure that parts of it are slowly (very, very slowly; geologically slowly) protruding. On this day, though, El Cap (as it is affectionately called) seems relaxed; it is the humans around me who are trying to shake off their tension. Shawn gazes at the looming cliff and remarks that looking at the top is making her *soooo nervous*, even as it's also clear that she can't seem to pull her eyes away.

Initially, Shawn seemed to have confidence in my ability to BASE jump after a few lessons, but by the time we met at Yosemite both of us understood that BASE jumping was not in my future. To me, the sport was just too scary. Not to mention that I am notoriously accident prone—at one point in my young life, I was a twenty-one-year-old training in the obscure sledding sport of luge at Lake Placid, with dreams of Olympic gold (and like most dreams, eventually thoroughly dashed); there, my nickname was "Crash." Enough said. Granted, I didn't feel good about this decision to forego BASE lessons. I wondered if this meant I was becoming, well, old. Still, I was here today because I wanted proximity to the magic. The very extremity of the sport, and that an older woman excelled at it, held some key to my quest, I was sure.

Shawn is a personal fitness trainer in her day job, though even this is a tame description of what she does: she is really an adventure trainer. Her website describes her career as "helping those who crave adventure but need some guidance . . . whether it is a mountain bike ride in the redwoods or skiing with the penguins in Antarctica." She tells me that her work is a response to the many people who say that they love her exploits and are living vicariously through her, something that repeatedly baffles her. She stares at each person and wonders, sometimes aloud to their faces, "What do *you* aspire to? What do *you* want to do? Just do it. Plan, research . . ."

Most of Shawn's clients are older women, drawn to her because they are—like many of us—dismayed at the way their bodies have changed. It's a particularly difficult part of aging for everyone, but for us women, who have for so long been taught to scrutinize our looks, it is especially destabilizing. Some reach for correctives—hyped emollients, plastic surgery, jade eggs, diet fads—and many, as in the case of Shawn's clients, a new exercise regime. But Shawn quickly noticed that there was more than some physical ideal missing from their lives. Even firm triceps and a high VO$_2$ max didn't seem to hold the answer. Many of her clients were off kilter in a deeper way, seeking something obscured by motherhood, by marriage, and by aging. They couldn't have articulated what beckoned, but it seemed to exist where bravery meets challenge meets the unknown. "I feel like women want adventure," Shawn tells me. "And they don't know how to get it."

Shawn trains her clients by bringing them up to speed physically, laying a foundation, then taking them on day expeditions. This progression—fitness first, then outdoor adventure—is not an accident. "When women start to feel stronger, and they look at themselves and they look different, then they start to see themselves differently," Shawn says. Her clients feel more in control of their lives as they meet goals and increase their energy, she adds, but they really begin to shed old notions of what they can and can't do once they are on mountains, in oceans, along trails. Early on, Shawn asks her clients, "What did you do when you were four and five? What did you do when you were ten? What were you doing activity-wise in high school?" This history of play as a kid allows Shawn to understand what adventures might speak to each woman, and it also reminds the woman of what she once loved to do but may no longer think of as possible. "I have one client who came to me for physical fitness. She told me her bike days were over. She just thought, I'm getting too old to do that. She was scared, and didn't think she had the strength anymore, and the skill set, and all that stuff. I'm like, 'You can totally ride your bike.'"

"And guess what," Shawn adds, smiling widely. "She's full-on mountain biking now."

Shawn herself was always an active kid. She was so active—always running, always moving quickly—that her parents sometimes harnessed her with a dog leash. Her parents gave her a boy's name because they had thought she was going to be a boy; when she wasn't they kept the name anyway. At four years old she became fascinated with the light that hung from the ceiling over a table in the living room. "I remember looking at that lamp constantly," she tells me. She noticed that if you bumped it, it would sway, reminding her of Tarzan and his vines from the television show she watched. "One day, I finally swung from that lamp. I fell on the marble table and broke it in half." It was her first BASE-like jump and she emerged, as she has from every jump since, completely unscathed.

The Indiana house she grew up in was at the end of a cul-de-sac. Beyond that was woods, and it was normal to roam those woods, and the neighborhood, unsupervised. "It looks so small now," Shawn says of the copse, but at the time it seemed like a huge, wild frontier. "I loved the adventure part. My friends and I called it 'exploring.' We'd say to each other, 'Let's go exploring!'" Her wilderness experience didn't extend much beyond that, though. Instead, Shawn excelled at team sports throughout her school years.

When Bruce took her canoeing on the Boundary Waters in Minnesota, "it was my first time doing something like that. Bruce [who is white] grew up doing all that kind of stuff with his dad and mom, but my family's never gone camping."

Sometime that first day they bumped a rock, and Shawn was pitched into the water. She thrashed around, panicked, and yelled for Bruce, who hadn't realized she had gone overboard. Finally, he heard her, looked back, and said calmly, "You know, you can stand up." The water, Shawn realized, was only as deep as her shins. "That's how frightened I was," she tells me now, laughing. "I was really afraid of everything. Wild-life, snakes, spiders, you name it."

This isn't a big surprise, given that the outdoors in this country has long been unwelcoming to people of color. For years, many national parks displayed FOR WHITES ONLY signs; in the South, these parks were only desegregated with the Civil Rights Act of 1964. The outdoor retail industry is also culpable: it marketed its wares exclusively to white consumers until only recently. In these ways, people of color have been systemically estranged from the wilderness, and "scrubbed from the mythical narrative of the Great American Outdoors," as a recent *New York Times* article notes. So it made sense when Shawn explained how anxious she used to be when she camped. At night, she wouldn't venture outside the tent without Bruce. "It was so dark!" she exclaims, and she had a fear of some-thing grabbing her—animals, humans, it wasn't clear. "When my parents went out for the night, they would always say, lock the door, don't open it for anybody, someone might steal you." Maybe that was also it, she muses, her subconscious harking back to childhood warnings.

Shawn is accustomed to being the only Black person in any situation—certainly she is one of the few, and one of the first, Black BASE jumpers. Story of her life, she tells me; there were hardly any Black kids in her private high school, and she was the only Black rower in college. Still, when she and Bruce travel to small towns, she often asks Bruce to go into a store without her, she'll stay in the van; it's just too exhausting to deal with the looks she gets from white people. What I gather from all this is that Shawn's extensive "exploring" is hard won. As a woman, as a Black woman. At first it may be difficult to square the outdoorsy BASE jumper of today with that frightened younger woman, but I am understanding that Shawn's many adventures come in spite of, or maybe because of, her fears. "I feel like it took me a while to figure out the world—and not be afraid of every little thing. Then I started to just venture off, to my own stuff."

When she was almost forty, Bruce gave her skydiving lessons for her birthday; like so many gifts between couples this was something he actually wanted to do himself. But Shawn thought it might be fun, went along with it, and sure enough, when she landed from her tandem jump she thought, That's so good. I want to do it again. Soon both she and Bruce were certified. After only twenty-five jumps, someone invited them to a bridge. Quickly she realized that while skydiving was fun, this was what she really wanted. Shawn became a BASE jumper.

"Why BASE over skydiving?" I ask. Fewer logistics? Less expense? Shawn pauses. Yes, partly that. But also, when you jump out of a plane, she says, there is the noise of the engine and the wind, and the air grabs you right away. In BASE jumping, "there is this *silence*." You don't reach terminal velocity immediately, so for three or four seconds after you step off the edge you are wrapped in absolute quiet. "Just silence," she repeats, almost reverent. "You feel so light." Then the air catches you. The roar begins. This is the signal to "go into your track," which means you form your body into a wing, with arms against sides and pointed toes.

Intrigued that just a few seconds can offer such reward, I ask Shawn to walk me through a BASE jump from the beginning. She explains that it starts with that step to the edge, also known as the "exit," and the pose: feet slightly apart, arms at her sides, head up. She glances at the parachute release handle to lock in where it is, then takes a few deep breaths to calm herself. She finds and focuses on a point far out in the distance; this keeps her stance tall, and her chest out—you want a big arch once in the air, she tells me—and then she mutters "Up and out, up and out" to herself a few times. It's important not to drop the head, she tells me, because all manner of bad things can happen, the worst being that the body inverts, the legs shoot skyward, and a deployed parachute tangles in the feet. Ready to jump now, she may spring from her knees or, to clear an object below, she may take a few steps back and do a running leap. But either way, she pushes herself forward, keeping that distant point in sight, throwing her arms outward to her sides as her feet leave the ground. At this point, many BASE jumpers shout "See ya!" as they disappear over the edge; this is not only an appropriately jaunty goodbye, but presumes a future in which the BASE jumper actually does encounter you later, to talk about her jump, have lunch, share a celebratory beer. This jump, the BASE jumper is saying, is like any other excursion we take in the world, and though this is patently untrue, it's a masterful stroke of propaganda toward moms, insurance agents, and naysayers.

Once airborne, Shawn begins to count. There is one, two, three seconds of that utter tranquility. A rush of air: she drops her head, pins arms to waist, points toes, tracks away. More counting—Shawn will have ten seconds of flying once off El Cap—then she deploys her pilot chute. When I ask about the emergency chute, in case this one doesn't open, she pauses and chuckles a little, then explains that there is no backup parachute, as there would not be time to deploy it (this is yet another detail that makes the sport so intimidating: no second chances). Other jumpers fly slightly differently; there isn't just one way, Shawn tells me. For instance, Bruce doesn't rely on counting, but determines when to deploy his chute from a spot on the cliff. When he jumps from an antenna he counts the lights he passes. Others just say they pull when the ground seems close, and Shawn laughs a little at the absurdity of that. "I stick to counting," she assures me.

Shawn and Bruce "go slick," which means that they wear normal clothes, not the fancy tracking suits that make a jumper more aerodynamic. Both also eschew the newer wingsuits that offer lift while in free fall and have introduced an even more dangerous permutation of BASE jumping called "proximity flying," where the goal is to stick as close to the terrain as possible. Jumping slick is old school. It often gets *Wowee* looks from younger BASE jumpers, who are certain that suits allow them more control, as well as speed away from the wall. But using suits of any kind entails a learning curve. "You have to practice in them, you can be surprised by them. We didn't want to go that route. If you know how to jump slick, you're fine," Shawn explains.

Bruce says that it's time to suss out the landing zone, so the four of us set off through shimmering aspens. As we walk, Shawn confesses that her palms have been sweating all day: on the steering wheel while driving, while arranging gear, and in her pockets right now. Bruce calls her the Reluctant BASE

Jumper, because routinely she can't sleep the night before an escapade and anxiety grips her right up until the moment her feet leave the edge and she is plummeting. For Shawn, the act of falling itself is not scary—it's the anticipation that gets her. No, it's not age, she tells me when I ask, it's always been like this. This is her normal rite of passage, pre-jump. Sure, every BASE jumper feels that shifting, often overlapping, line between anxiety and exhilaration; for Shawn, though, these nerves are epic. It's better if she's jumping simultaneously with Bruce and Jimmy. Bombs away on the count of three, and that's all it takes, she tells me—they are in the air, tracking away from each other. She knows this doesn't make sense; there's nothing Bruce or Jimmy can do if something goes wrong. Still, she doesn't hesitate—on *three* she is airborne. But jumping without them is completely different. She has stood on a cliff stammer-stepping for almost a half hour. She sent me the video that documented this: in it, Shawn looks up at the sky, down at her feet, over the edge. Let's be clear—the whole scenario looks intimidating. There is dense fog. It's very cold. Below (far, far) lies greenery and a river, seen only inter-mittently and as a hazy splotch. Jimmy counts down for her—3, 2, 1—but she can't get herself off the edge. Her face is fixed in a half smile; she wrings her hands once or twice. But never does she turn to the other BASE jumpers, who can be heard on the video impatiently awaiting their turn, and say "I can't do it" or "I'm so scared," or offer teary apologies. Instead she talks to herself—"I'm going to do it, I'm going to do it"—or to Jimmy—"Is this the longest anyone has ever taken at the edge?" (yes). Finally, she does jump, and she's ecstatic after-ward. "It was great," she tells the camera, beaming, "Let's do it again."

So how does she get herself off the edge? When I ask, it's hard for her to explain. Perhaps it's the shame of keeping others waiting. Or she is able to momentarily offline the voices that tell her that jumping is ridiculous. Mostly, she tells me, it's a simple cost-benefit analysis—she knows how much she will regret a missed opportunity to fly. The ever-present four-year-old wins, the innate understanding that it's Tarzan who has all the fun, not passive Jane. Once she's in the air, she explains, the anxiety is gone. Completely and utterly vanished. Suddenly it's the best thing in the world to be here, that reverberating silence, that falling toward earth. Even when things don't go right, like the time she jumped and immediately somersaulted: "The thing about me is that I get really calm when things get hairy, so I said, Oh, I'm doing a flip," Shawn remembers. "I came out of it, and tracked away." Now here she is, soon to leap from a three-thousand-foot face while knowing that she will be terrified at the edge, that it will mean lining up all that she loves about BASE jumping against all that tells her it's a big mistake. That's the math: multiple weeks of planning, forty-eight hours of sweating palms, an arduous six-hour hike equals three seconds of stillness, a ten-second free fall, and less than two total minutes of exhilaration in the air.

Not to be forgotten: so much of the BASE jump adventure also involves walking around for hours in the breathtaking scenery of a prized national park. We hike through rumpled meadows, planning escape routes. We veer into wooded glens, discussing in whispers the best place to hide get-away bicycles. We scan binoculars along the rock face to clock phantom glide paths with the earnest enthusiasm of bird-watchers. Glancing right and left to make sure we aren't seen, we step toward the sand bars near the river to assess a landing zone. Finally, the plan is solid. The dawn jump is scrapped; instead, Shawn, Bruce, and Jimmy will hike all the next day, arriving at the top of El Cap right before sunset. I am fresh off a knee surgery, so the six-hour hike up, not to mention the hike back down again, is impossible. I'm still part of the adventure, though: I'm in one of the most beautiful places in the world. I'm wandering meadows and trails among aspens, learning about the tricks of shedding parachute rigs and ski pants while running to a hidden bicycle. I'm offering my small assistance to this caper, which qualifies me as "ground crew" or, perhaps more accurately, "accomplice."

Honestly, this adventure today is my first real step into nature in a while. I confess: for months I had been in a lethargy brought on by the early days of the pandemic, which had then deepened once summer wildfire smoke began to thicken the skies. Routinely I looked out from our hilltop window and was unable to see a skyline. The houses just a block away were blurry and unformed. I felt claustrophobic, depressed. As the smoke cleared, my mood did not, and I couldn't rouse myself to go outside, even though I knew it was the antidote. Now, as terms like "deploy," "off heading," and "burble" float like random leaves around me, I feel myself quickening among the brilliant meadows, the swaying grasses, and the soft wing-beats of warm air. I may not be BASE jumping, but I am exhilarated and animated nevertheless.

At 4:30 P.M. I position myself in a field facing El Cap. My job is to look for rangers; nobody wants to jump in full view of them, which is why BASE escapades are usually done in the dead of night, under cover of darkness, lit only by a moon and some hope. This seems treacherous, given uneven terrain and spearlike trees, but Shawn assures me that jumping with any daylight, even twilight daylight, is much more dangerous, because the threat of being seen and caught is so high. Summoning all I know about lookouts from action movies, I find a place to sit and watch without attracting any attention. I scan the road. All clear. The meadow has filled with visitors eager to catch the alpenglow, or climbers with binoculars who make last checks on friends shimmying skyward, who can be seen as tiny, dark specks even without magnification. I alternately swing my own binoculars from the looming rock to the far ends of the encircling road. Nothing is out of the ordinary. At 5:30 P.M., I key my radio. Like all good rascals and skulkers, we're using code in case anyone is monitoring our channel. "Hanging out waiting for you guys," I say, to indicate I am in position. I add, "And Frank isn't here yet," to tell them there are no rangers in sight. The sun seems to spark as it sinks toward the mountain range. Bruce radios back. "We're leaving the hotel in twenty," he says. "See you soon."

El Cap is half in shadow when I finally see a tiny form step up to the rim. Shawn! I imagine her eyes resolutely fixed on a point across the valley, her low incantation of "up and out, up and out." Thirty seconds pass. I know that Shawn's biggest fear is that she will not get herself off the edge in time for Jimmy and Bruce to get film footage of their jump in the fading light. As she stands there, a miniature silhouette of bravery and hesitation, my own heart speeds up. I check my watch again—a minute has gone by. This will be a long one, and why not? BASE jumping is terrifying. But suddenly she is dropping. You don't realize how huge El Cap is until a minuscule human is falling in front of it. I gasp. She is falling so fast, and so far, that I only have time to imagine her triumphant smile, that cocoon of silence, and then a blue parachute pops open with the surprise and suddenness of a magician's flower.

There is a collective gasp as those in the field realize a BASE jumper has suddenly manifested against the colossal wall. Shawn's canopy dips and turns right, to whoops and scattered applause. I can almost hear everyone around me whispering, "Holy moly, that guy has balls." What would they think if they knew that they were watching not a swaggering young buck, but a fifty-two-year-old woman? Shawn drops behind the tree line, flying toward the designated landing zone. Bruce and Jimmy jump now, two tiny teardrops against the dark wall. Their chutes unfurl, one with a loud *thwack*. The audience members clap again. Then the two of them drop quickly out of sight.

And now it's over. I haven't seen the actual landings, but I am sure it has all gone off without a hitch. I'm grinning from ear to ear. I gather my things, jump on my Onewheel, head to my car (finally, with Shawn present at the gate, I was able to bring my car into the park), drive to the meeting point. I wait for their triumphant return. And wait. And wait. It gets dark. The stars come out.

Finally, I accept it: something has gone wrong.

All three had landed in the right spot, exactly as planned. But within moments Bruce saw people in brown running at them from all directions. It was like some bad cop show, the hapless rangers staggering as they negotiated the deep sand near the river while yelling for the BASE jumpers to stay where they were—"Don't move! Stop!" How had they arrived so quickly? The only explanation: they had been lying in wait. A climber at the top of El Cap, Bruce later figures, perhaps that guy who asked for water and wondered what they were doing? But in this moment the melee was only just registering. "Don't run," Bruce told Shawn. Jimmy either didn't hear Bruce or simply took his chances. He booked before the rangers got a good look at him, and when the rangers asked about a third person, Bruce and Shawn shrugged and feigned confusion.

The park jail was closed due to the pandemic, so Bruce and Shawn were spared a night in the clink. But a formal ticket was written up. They were frisked next to a car with flashing police lights. Their gear was confiscated. They'd cooperated and that was good, the ranger said, but mercy was not on the agenda, and they'd have to show up in court. "It's illegal?" Shawn asked at one point, trying to play dumb, but the rangers weren't having it. "No aerial endeavors in the park!" they barked. Neither Bruce nor Shawn has ever been arrested before. Now it will be many months before they get their canopies and harnesses back, if ever. I drive to pick them up.

Where's Jimmy? Finally, I receive a text from him. He's hiding under a log, he'll make for the road, can we come with the car? He drops a pin from his phone to show his location. When we find him it's almost nine o'clock. His story is breathless, hilarious: he had hightailed it to the river, throwing away his gear as he ran. Goodbye ski pants, goodbye sunglasses, goodbye backpack. He'd also discarded the cameras, tucking one in the nook of a tree, another at the base of a berm, in the hopes that they wouldn't be found and used as evidence. He'd splashed across the water, then jammed himself under a fallen tree. He heard the rangers crashing around in the brush nearby, but they never found him. Did they find the gear? We venture back out into the night, trying to match the terrain around us with the accounting of his mad dash. We wade through the river and clomp up the hill, shining our headlamps. We don't find everything, but we find some of it, and the next day the rest is procured. Jimmy has been lucky, Bruce and Shawn have not.

But me? I feel awash in luck. And elation. I wasn't the badass BASE jumper, but I have spent two days in the beautiful outdoors, party to the adventure. The wildfires erasing towns and mountains and wildlife have been forgotten. The pandemic, with its horrors of illness and uncertainty, is on the back burner. Even my depression has receded, replaced by adrenaline and wonder.

There's only one thing I would have had otherwise: I wish I'd seen the rangers' faces. What were they thinking when they realized that the flying daredevil-ruffian in their custody was in fact a woman in her fifties, a kindergarten teacher, a mother, a *grandmother*? As each ranger clocked the incongruous perp before them, weren't they also unconsciously trying to square their beliefs about older women, and coming up short? In that moment, surely, a narrative shifted just a little. A chink of negative messaging fell away, like a small bit of rock from the face of El Cap itself.

And then, in my imagination at least, word quickly reaches the entrance gate where I had only recently glided by on my Onewheel: *A fifty-two-year-old woman has BASE jumped off El Cap. Older than my mom!* I think of those rangers taking that in, perplexed at how, twice in a week, older ladies have been seen doing something a little wacko. "Must be a full moon or something," someone might say, chuckling derisively. But not everyone. At least a few will realize that yes, one older woman is a fluke. But two? That is something verging on a truth they can't quite grasp.

One more thing: the case adjudicating these rapscallion ways is still pending as of this writing. Shawn, a menace only to our sense of cultural order and not much more, waits for her day in court, hoping for leniency or even a change in park rules. Her BASE gear resides in some moldy evidence cage; she hasn't been able to jump in over a year.

I thought I had come to Yosemite to indulge my curiosity for a sport that had circled the periphery of my vision for years. I was also interested in how older women came to Shawn to help them change their bodies into sleek, younger machines. Instead, Shawn has made it clear that it's not enough to cut fat and add a few muscles—that it is adventure that many of us crave. And there is something more. Watching Shawn has been inspirational—an overused word, perhaps, but don't let that undermine its power. As an identical twin I know the importance of looking to someone else for guidance. I believe deeply in role models. Because it's not just the young rangers who don't have a clue about our potential; we don't, either. Therefore, we need templates in our life. We need to see our possible selves in someone else's grand exploits. "You cannot be what you cannot see," said the civil rights activist Marian Wright Edelman, and she is correct.

As amazing a role model as she is, Shawn will probably dismiss us if we marvel too much at her daring. She'll murmur, dismayed, that everyone should just follow suit. Sorry, Shawn, but most of us will never be BASE jumpers. It is uniquely dangerous, terrifying, and often illegal. But it still has a lesson to teach us. We can be quickened by Shawn's skill and courage, enlivened by her exploits. Like her adventure clients, we want to change our minds about ourselves. We want to marvel, to dream, and then we want to scuff our feet at our own edge, spooked and uncertain. What is that edge? We don't yet know, perhaps, but now we will look for it. We will then stand at that edge whispering self-help incantations to urge ourselves off, the minutes ticking by. With mentors like Shawn, we will take a tentative step, then leap into our own wide, open sky.

3

Buoyancy Matters

Age is no barrier. It's a limitation you put on your mind.

—JACKIE JOYNER-KERSEE, SIXTY, OLYMPIAN IN TRACK
AND FIELD FROM 1984 TO 1998

I n 1958, researchers at the National Institutes of Health decided to investigate the fundamentals of growing old. In particular, they wanted to understand why some people aged well and others struggled physically and mentally in their later years. To do this, they inaugurated the Baltimore Longitudinal Study of Aging, which followed thousands of people from their twenties onward, assessing them every two years with questionnaires and physical exams, continuing the research after death with autopsies. During the autopsies, one of the conditions the scientists evaluated was brain health.

Here they found an astounding link: those with negative views on aging (gleaned from the questionnaires administered at the outset of the study) "showed significantly steeper hippocampal volume loss and significantly greater accumulation of neurofibrillary tangles and amyloid plaques." In other words, these people had physically deteriorating brains. There was, the scientists realized, a statistical correlation between thinking of aging as infirmity and disease and fulfillment of those views. Ditto for cardiovascular health: those who equated aging with frailty and illness had twice the chance of a fatal heart attack, and at an earlier age, too.

Even more significant, the opposite is also true—an empowering view of aging leads to a longer, healthier life. Researcher Becca Levy examined the Baltimore data and found that those who "held positive age beliefs from the outset went on to experience 30% better memory scores in old age than their peers with negative age beliefs." As she writes in her book *Breaking the Age Code*, Levy also looked at the Ohio Longitudinal Study on Aging and Retirement, and realized that those with an optimistic attitude lived an average of seven and a half years longer than their more defeatist peers. Ultimately Levy came to the astounding conclusion that when it comes to longevity, one's perspective is not just a significant factor, it is *the most significant* factor. It matters even more than variables like one's physical health, education, or financial situation.

These studies reveal an important truth: aging does not have to be a dispiriting spiral. If we shift our mindset, our later years can be a time of exploration, adventure, and joy. Finding that positive mindset can be difficult, however. Aging sucks, we are told constantly by the media, by the job market, by dating apps. We're stunned to be no longer young, not even middle-aged, but officially "older," or even, if we are to be honest, old. Yet our experience of being fifty-, sixty-, seventy-, or eighty-something does not match that definition of "old" that we solidified as kids observing the adults around us, which we tucked away, appalled, years ago, only to face it now, rife with its faults and misconceptions.

It isn't just our own preconceived notions that dog us. For women especially, the societal messages around aging continue to be disheartening. Men are seen as distinguished, sexy, and powerful as their years advance, and for inspiration they get James Bond villains, all fiery-eyed and trying to blow up the world. Sure, these curmudgeonly role models ultimately die at the hands of 007, but they are always unrepentant, shouting whole paragraphs of last words and banging on their chests before the final moment. Villains, yes, but living out their post-fifty years with outsize appetites and chutzpah, until a buzz saw or a bullet exits them with great fanfare stage left.

In contrast, a woman growing old is the most boring movie ever, a bland narrative where the main character battles—what? Increasing invisibility. A loss of relevance. Hand-to-hand combat with . . . one's own insignificance. Movies, advertisements, books, and the indifferent expressions of those younger than us all scream the same message—women of a certain age have little to offer, and therefore are no longer of cultural importance. We grew up believing that. Now we have arrived at this moment, and we believe it of ourselves. No wonder most of us begin this important expedition—our own inevitable aging—with the emotional equivalent of a ratty sleeping bag and a leaking tent.

Louise Wholey doesn't seem to have heard the news that aging is difficult, diminishing, and a total bore. At age eighty, she can still hoist her scuba tank onto her back from a sitting position if she maneuvers it right. Right now, she stands, then penguins around to peer out toward the ocean, and I follow her gaze, clutching my new fins and mask. I have just recertified in scuba diving after a long absence from the water (twenty years); compared to Louise, who has six hundred dives under her belt, I am a mere baby bird, scooting to the edge of the nest. "You're the expert," I tell her when she suggests that our dive follow the jetty wall, taking in the fish that hide in the rocks and the kelp that sways along its edge. "Oh, I'm no expert," she responds. "There is always something new to learn." This is why I'm here today: I want to figure out the secret behind Louise's expansive attitude, and how it links to the gumption that keeps her diving long after most people decades younger have hung up their masks and tanks. In other words, is outdoor adventure at a later age not just the result of a positive attitude toward getting older, but actually the integral gateway to *achieving* that positive attitude?

I have white hair, range about 5'7", Caucasian. This is how Louise described herself in a text so I would recognize her when I pulled my car into our Monterey, California, meeting place—though if she had written *the Person Older Than Everyone Else*, it would have been just as helpful. There are many divers milling around this pretty little beach park today, but they are almost exclusively under forty. Still, it's impossible to me that Louise is actually eighty years old. Despite her wrinkled skin, etched in the manner of someone who has been outdoors her whole life, she moves with the short steps and bowed legs of a soccer player. When she stands, the curve of her upper back that sometimes comes with aging reminds me of a slouchy teenager at the mall. I wonder: When she dons her heavy scuba equipment and people suddenly realize how old she is, what do they say? "The typical reaction is 'NO. You're not eighty,'" she says. "Or"—and here she feigns horror—"'You're *eighty*?'"

I laugh and nod, and think, Sounds about right. Then I ask if she is proud of that mixture of surprise and admiration so evident on their faces. "I would be," I tell her. I mean, she's representing all older women in that instance, and overturning prejudgments about what we can and cannot do. "That's a thrill, right?" She thinks about this for a moment. "I don't have an attitude about age. It's just something you carry with you. You can't escape it." She shrugs. "I don't think much about it, I guess."

Louise's curious indifference to getting older is not exactly the same as a positive view on aging, but it still makes her the embodiment of what can happen when you are free of negative stereotypes and diminished expectations. Certainly, there is something uniquely defiant about scuba diving in these particular waters at eighty years old. This part of the Pacific Ocean is always frigid (on this summer day, it is fifty degrees). The visibility can drop to almost nothing. When the wind picks up, there is a swell on entry from the beach that can knock you down. Oh, did I mention the shark attack? A swimmer was bitten by a great white two days ago, shutting down some of the coastline. Louise texted me about it, lamenting the potential beach closure, but not the lurking shark. I think the text was also a courtesy—she was unperturbed, but perhaps I might not want to dive? (I did.)

Fully clad in our gear, we make our way along the grass that overlooks the ocean, past other wet-suit-skinned humans who have already begun to gather in earnest, so that from afar it might look like mating season among seals. This is a popular place for scuba divers and has remained open despite the attack. Still, as we reach the wide stone stairs that lead to a small sandy beach, a sign affixed to sawhorses shouts, REALLY? YOU WANT TO GO IN THE WATER? WHY THE HELL ARE YOU THAT DUMB? (It actually reads, WARNING SHARK ATTACK OCCURRED . . . ENTER WATER AT YOUR OWN RISK, with a photo of two shark fins cutting through ocean swell. But there are the words, and then there is the way my wife would have interpreted it.) We negotiate the stairs, and as we lumber to the water's edge, Louise mentions that sharks, even the ferocious whites, are unlikely to attack divers—they usually hit victims on the surface, mistaking them for a hapless seal. Humans—the two of us, is what she's really saying—aren't appetizing for sharks. I'm not concerned, and I tell her so as we wade through the break. I know the odds of being bitten are minuscule, and anyway there are at least fifty divers who will soon be out today, from whom the shark can choose. We float, affix our masks to our heads, and then Louise gives the thumbs-down—not a commentary on my diving skills so far, just the signal to descend. From now on we will be using hand gestures to speak: to communicate that one is fine, the OK sign is flashed; a thumbs-up is a signal to ascend (if you, like me, tend to try to tell your diving companion that you are

OK by jauntily flipping the thumbs-up underwater, well, things get a little confusing); and so on.

When Louise began diving in 1962, upon the urging of a college boyfriend, the sport was just getting popular; Jacques Cousteau was well known, the television show *Sea Hunt*, about a retired navy frogman and his underwater heroics battling all manner of villain, was a huge hit. Still, you had to glue together your own wet suit using pieces of neoprene, and the breathing apparatus was quaintly called an "aqualung." There was no buoyancy control vest, and if you needed to float on the surface you might blow a few breaths into an inflatable neck ring that resembled a child's toy. Underwater, you simply had to fin wildly. Today Louise wears more state-of-the-art gear: a buoyancy control wing, a tank of nitrox, and a dry suit to protect her from the cold, which requires extra training and many hours in the water to master.

Louise was clear from the start that my basic certification was just a "license that now lets you learn how to dive." Even something as simple seeming as keeping oneself off the seafloor takes hours of instruction and practice. Certainly, descending with slow grace, while clearing ears to adjust for pressure and chomping tightly on the mouthpiece as one's brain slowly grasps the strange reality of breathing underwater, is not easy. True to form, I make my way to the bottom looking like that drowned body during the opening credits of a Netflix thriller—lit by a ray of light from above, arms out, feet splayed, tumbling slowly. Naturalist Barry Lopez writes that diving is a form of "intense, amorous contact" with Mother Nature, and he is correct, but that includes the awkward groping and inadvertent teeth-clashing of adolescents in a romantic embrace. I hit the sand butt first instead of what Louise does, which is hover, fins down, then turn slowly horizontal and begin a swim just inches from the seafloor, never once touching it. Louise once took a weeklong intensive course on buoyancy alone, she later explains, with the goal being mastery of "neutral buoyancy." This is the balance between the water and one's own density, allowing a diver to suspend herself exactly where she wants at any given moment. While a beginner opts for maniacally kicking with her fins or hammering down on the valve that diverts air from the tank into her vest for more underwater flotation, someone proficient uses variables as subtle as her own breath, as well as just the right titration of tank air at just the correct time. Neutral buoyancy can't be attained by fighting or flailing. It is the ultimate in equilibrium, a symmetry of forces, a gentle kinetic dance. Which is why at this moment I look like a toddler unable to control her limbs, and Louise is slowly undulating out of my sight.

Diving with a landlubber is a departure from Louise's usual routine. Much of her time under the ocean is spent in the service of citizen science, often for a conservation nonprofit called Reef Check: counting fish, measuring kelp, surveying the rocky outcrops. (Her husband, Jim, no longer gets into cold water, but she often partners up with her daughter, who is also an experienced diver and volunteer.) Scuba diving for science is not just taxing; it can be tedious, with its requisite repetition and attention to minutiae. But Louise assures me that for her, "it's always interesting and challenging." When Louise assesses kelp health, for instance, she has to count the stipes that grow from each main stem, or hold-fast, as it is called. They can number up to one hundred, and even more than that, in a healthy plant. It's often difficult to keep up the count, because the kelp is "swaying back and forth in the current and you're swaying back and forth," she explains; I imagine it's like someone pushing on your pencil as you attempt to add up a very long grocery receipt. While Reef Check mandates an annual refresher of new species and new survey techniques, it's up to the volunteer diver to keep up skills such as trim and buoyancy and Louise takes this seriously, which means she's a valued underwater volunteer. She spreads this expertise around: when it's not Reef Check, it's work with the Giant Giant Kelp Restoration Project (G2KR), or she's donning her gear for Clean Up the Lake to pick up garbage from Lake Tahoe, where the water is routinely forty-three degrees and the volunteers recently surfaced almost three hundred pounds of refuse in just one day. "It's diving with a purpose," she tells me. "I guess that in my little way, I want to make the world a little better."

Today the visibility is a murky fifteen or so feet, and it soon drops below that. The effect is of a slightly menacing but beautiful fairy tale forest, where dark shadows resolve into rocks covered in orange anemones as you get closer, and the kelp looks like deformed trees behind which a gingerbread house or a monster might lurk. It's quiet except for the roar of my own breath on exhale, and everything moves in slow motion—the gentle sway of stipe, the dance of anemone arms. Huge starfish drape themselves on rocks, and now and then a fish as large as my hand darts by. At one point, a whole school envelops me, and it feels as if I am shooting through space among asteroids. The ocean can be so strange and beautiful as to play games with one's head (also there is the real danger of nitrogen buildup, which mimics the effects of drunkenness), so that at times I have to remind myself that I am a diver, underwater, breathing through a tube, and that I am OK. (OK sign here.) Mostly, though, I keep a close eye on Louise. I don't want to lose her in the murk, because it would be embarrassing, for one, and also unnerving to be suddenly alone in this dark and muffled world.

My scuba experience before this entailed only a handful of real dives, unless you count being a rescue diver while a firefighter with the San Francisco Fire Department, where I worked for almost fourteen years, which I don't. I'm not being coy here. I don't even tell Louise of this background, because it might signal that I know more about this sport than I actually do. Diving in the San Francisco Bay for dead bodies or tossed guns sounds tricky, but it requires little more than steely nerves. The water is cold but not frigid, and it isn't deep. There is little surge. The visibility is nil, however, and you learn to descend the fifteen feet or so, stop at what seems like the muddy bottom, then descend farther into three feet of viscous silt. Only then do you begin the search, one hand holding a rope that leads to the surface and guides you, while the other arm sweeps slowly back and forth. As brave as we pretended to be, nobody really liked the idea of coming upon the decayed flesh, the tattered clothing, the bloated limbs, the vacant eye sockets. (For some reason, the fact that eyeballs were a delicacy for marauding fish always stuck in my mind.) During my career as a firefighter I never actually found a body—by the time my crew was called, it had always been swept away by tides and currents. But we dove anyway, contending with shopping carts, car tires, and strange wooden pylons, none of which we could actually see. Also, tiny crabs would scuttle over our wet suits as we slowly finned along the bottom, like a million tiny fingers. This took some getting used to, but once the initial startle was mastered, it wasn't as disturbing as it sounds. Part of me found it comforting that there were benign, excitable creatures with me in that thick, muddy dark, and I took their effervescent darts and scratches as proof that the normal world still existed above. All in all, this kind of diving resembled fighting a fire more than scuba diving, with the pitch black, the household objects in the way, and the singular focus of finding a human, in this case a dead one.

Today, I can see everything around me, and there is no particular goal but to enjoy it. Here, the intricate structure of a tiny barnacle. There, the scuttle of a small crustacean. I'm especially intrigued with a finger-sized creature that looks like sand until it skitters away from my shadow. There, the translucence of kelp, and there, the languid droop of a sea cucumber. Scuba diving, I am realizing, is actually a relaxing activity, something always done slowly. One breathes slowly, descends and ascends slowly, and swims slowly. We fin (slowly) along the wall, and Louise points to strange creatures that cling to the rocks and sometimes to the kelp stipes. She tries to use her slate to write down each name, but the underwater pencil is broken, which is fine, as I'm happy to observe nature free of proper nouns. Instead I just gape at these unknowable existences beneath the ocean, a whole *Umwelt* that humans can't fully grasp. At one point, a bird flies by and this delights me—a bird! Underwater! I have seen birds disappear from the surface to fish, but never thought about what happened once they dove. Turns out, they torpedo down, then jet along the bottom, feet churning, neck outstretched. This one blurs by, and I manage to laugh through the regulator in my mouth without choking.

As the dive progresses, the surge picks up, and I struggle to keep from crashing into Louise or an unsuspecting limpet. I am also beginning to shiver. (Unlike Louise, I wear a simple wet suit, which doesn't keep me as warm as a dry suit would.) Once or twice a looming dark shadow threatens to resolve into an underwater monster (shark?), but I talk my mind out of it. It's a rock, I tell myself, or kelp. And sure enough, it is.

Louise has explained that her dive missions sometime entail wholesale slaughter, specifically of the sea urchins that now crowd the ocean floor. The murder of urchins seems an unlikely pastime for an eighty-year-old, but Louise describes the "smashing" technique with little emotion, except to add that the arthritis in her hand acts up after a while. She'll kill hundreds at a time, and without regret. At first I am taken aback at Louise's matter-of-fact tone, but soon realize that from the point of view of an ocean lover she is acting more in self-defense than as an abject serial killer. Urchins, I come to learn, have been quickly multiplying for over a decade after their main predator, the sunflower sea star, contracted a wasting disease, probably from the warming oceans. Now unchecked, the voracious urchins eat huge amounts of kelp, which in turn leaves invertebrates without food, fish without protection, and the oceans without a carbon dioxide filter. Divers like Louise wield hammers with pick ends to methodically annihilate the urchins, hoping to clear areas and allow for kelp growth. It seems like a fanciful effort, another clumsy human intervention to right a human wrong, but Louise says that after just one year of smashing there is one hundred square meters of nearby ocean floor where the urchins have been cleared and the kelp is rejuvenating. "Just a year ago, it was an urchin barren, just urchins and rock but little else—no kelp at all." Today she describes it as lush with plant and fish life. The science is not yet clear on who will eventually win the battle, but studies are being done. "It's not like I am killing a healthy animal doing good things for the habitat," Louise says, perhaps clocking my slightly shocked vegan face. "I don't have any issue helping to bring the ocean back into balance."

Volunteer workers like Louise experience many benefits, studies have found. Offering one's time to count stipes or pick up trash provides much needed relief for the environment, yes, but it also provides benefits for the volunteer herself, including countering the feeling of being superfluous that often comes with age. By diving for science, Louise remains vital and productive, as well as intimately involved in the present even as it means coming face-to-face under the ocean with the precarious state of our earth above. Similarly, the journalist and explorer Tara Roberts writes about the sometimes excruciating, sometimes jubilant, always enlightening experience of becoming an "underwater archeology advocate" with a nonprofit called Diving with a Purpose. Along with other African American scuba divers of all ages, she surveys the sunken wrecks of forgotten slave ships. Salvaged are not just gut-wrenching artifacts like shackles, but also the more complete history of a ship's ghastly journey, allowing the volunteers to play an important part in fully excavating our nation's past. The effect on them is profound, Roberts tells us. The work is difficult and traumatic, but "there's something extraordinary about Black people saying, I am going to go out and find my own history, and I'm going to shape the stories that are told about it," she explains. The group is full of young divers, but also participating are divers over fifty, and they are no doubt key to the group's continuing successes: when outdoor adventure in the sphere of citizen science is difficult both technically and psychologically, older people bring an emotional sturdiness and big-picture sensibility vital to the health of the project and of its participants.

I tap my finger on my air gauge and twirl my finger, indicating that I've reached the turn-around point on my tank. We begin to swim back the way we came. The visibility has dropped even more, but I can still see the bright purple of the dreaded urchins. The movement of the water against the jetty has intensified, and I'm fully shivering now; within a short span of time the dive has tipped from engrossing to uncomfortable—not uncommon in these difficult waters. I'm amazed that Louise does multiple dives a day, sometimes many times a week.

It's worth mentioning here that scuba can be expensive. It requires a lot of equipment (rented or bought), and sometimes boats. But its close relative, snorkeling, is pretty cheap. All that is needed to snorkel is a mask, and fins if you want to get fancy. Snorkeling offers a similar peek into a strange and beautiful world, and with it a sense of venturing into the elements. You are still communing with the ocean. You are still immersing yourself in the vagaries of nature. You may not get the admiring feedback that Louise gets, because scuba belongs squarely in the realm of Navy SEALS, while snorkeling evokes emerald bays and holidays. Nevertheless you are on an adventure with each fish you wonder at and each dark mound that you swim toward, uncertain if it will be monster or rock.

Louise may not think much about age these days, but I wonder what ideas she held when she was young. "Young people don't think about getting old," she tells me with the same matter-of-fact attitude that allows her to kill those urchins and that has guided her years of work in, no surprise here, particle physics at first, then computer engineering. Okay, how about as you aged, I persist—what views did you have about aging in your forties, fifties? She thinks for a moment. Then the scientist in her steps up again with empirical evidence. "Well, when I got into my sixties, I started doing one-hundred-mile runs." She thinks a little more. "When I turned seventy I completed the triple crown extended of biking," which entails successfully peddling five two-hundred-mile races in a year, plus a volunteer stint at one of the bike races, too. "On my seventieth birthday I finished the last of the 248 peaks in the Sierras. I'd been working on that ever since I got to California in 1969 . . . Does that answer your question?"

Yes, it does. Louise, it seems, just goes about her life, unhindered by stereotypes or societal expectations (or as it were, societal *un*-expectations). Sure, one of her knees has been replaced and the other needs it. Sure, she has a strained shoulder and arthritis. Sure, she's eighty. But who cares?

Louise's mindset about aging reflects research done in 1979 by a scientist named Ellen Langer. Interested in the way our subconscious beliefs guide us, Langer convinced eight men in their seventies to stay together in a house for five days. The house was a time machine, decorated only with artifacts from twenty years before—from the newspapers delivered every day, to the shows from that era that played on the small black-and-white television, to the music on the old-timey radio. In addition, there were no mirrors to jolt the seventy-year-olds to reality; they were instead surrounded by photos of their younger faces. Completing the time machine effect was the mandate that the men and the researchers who interacted with them speak only of events from two decades earlier, and to do so in the present tense. Langer was clear on this point: she didn't want the men to merely remember their prime from their current vantage point, she wanted to thoroughly immerse them in a world that treated them as if they were *actually twenty years younger*. She theorized that if they "put their mind in an earlier time," their bodies would follow. Meanwhile a control group of men of similar age also lived together for five days; they were encouraged to wax nostalgic, but otherwise they lived completely in their seventy-year-old present.

When the Counterclockwise study, as it came to be known, was over, the men who had been treated as if they were younger showed such marked improvement that the researchers could hardly believe the numbers; Langer later said the results "sounded like Lourdes." Postures straightened, flexibility improved, grip strength shot up, and cognitive function sharpened. Volunteers asked to assess photographs of the men even incorrectly pegged them as much younger *after* the study than before.

Dr. Langer knew that sixteen male-only subjects did not make for a conclusive scientific study, but it nevertheless began the reckoning: Dr. Langer saw that there was a powerful connection between mind and body. She realized that cues, called *primes*, act as a lens through which information is filtered, and the beliefs triggered by these primes can be so powerful as to change our very physiology. If this is true, she argues, shouldn't we pick as many positive primes as possible?

With its attendant feelings of accomplishment, community, physical vigor, and experiences of beauty, scuba is a powerful lens through which to fortify one's sense of self. Snorkeling works, too: Suspended in a new medium, explorers of a strange world, momentarily exhilarated, how could we not be opened up to the idea of new possibilities about ourselves? And there is more: Doesn't outdoor adventure like this immerse us, just as those men in Dr. Ellen Langer's study were immersed, in the experience of someone younger? But it's not about actually being younger. It's about claiming those aspects of physical vitality, novelty, exhilaration, agency, and adventure for ourselves, at this age, right now.

Louise tells me that it was her doctor who ultimately changed her outlook. "I was complaining about some injury I had, [and he said,] 'Louise, the only difference between you and an eighteen-year old is that you blame these things on age.' That completely changed my view from one that says aging is debilitating to one that says age does not matter."

So thoroughly has Louise adopted this particular lens, or "prime," as researchers Langer and Levy would put it, that now she seems outright baffled by my questions. "Look, life doesn't end at forty or fifty," she says. "And you have a choice. You can be a couch potato, or you can decide that whatever ails you is insignificant." Even as she's had to forsake rock climbing (hurts her hand), cut back on long ski expeditions (knees), and slow down her hikes (ditto), she continues to dive. "The ocean is supportive," she says.

Now on dry land, I ask Louise how I did. "You seemed comfortable," she manages, pointedly not mentioning that underwater I am an ungainly amalgam of jerking limbs, constantly trying not to crash into the rocks, working hard and sometimes unsuccessfully to keep from flipping on my back like an unfortunate insect, often dog-paddling wildly to avoid bumping into her. Not mentioned, also: as we were swimming on the surface back toward the beach, one of my fins fell off. Caught on a fishing line cast from shore, it unsnapped, slid from my foot, and sank. Then it lay on the bottom, fifteen feet below, the slowly shifting sand making it look as if it were winking at me. I suppressed a momentary panic. My fin is gone! Then, in the next second, I realized I could just put the breathing apparatus back into my mouth and retrieve it. With one fin, I awkwardly kicked down to the other, prodigal fin. I was neither underwater bird nor sleek sea creature, just an anxious, discombobulated human, but I reached it. As I surfaced again, relieved, I thought, Well, that wasn't worth panicking about. Mastery of neutral buoyancy beckoned, that ability to balance not just the physical forces that keep us from being exactly where we want to be, but the mental ones that jerk us off kilter, so that we are gaping at the one dropped fin and thinking, Whelp, there goes that thing, sorry. No, silly, guess what. You are fully equipped to retrieve it. Mindset, even in this small instance, mattered, and once I groped for the empowering *you can*, it turned out that, yes, I could.

Now, our tanks at our feet and lunch beckoning, Louise and I take a final look at the ocean, and Louise mentions that kelp grows two feet a day. This sounds hopeful, and I say that maybe kelp will win; despite the odds, it will grow and grow and grow, insistent, persistent, defying expectations, and Louise nods, *of course it will.*

BODY

4

Just Move

Go outside, often, sometimes in wild places.
Bring friends or not. Breathe.

—FLORENCE WILLIAMS, AGE FIFTY-FIVE, AUTHOR,
THE NATURE FIX

D ot Fisher-Smith and I are on a walk, and at this moment she is cutting across someone's suburban front yard. She has already told me she doesn't like sidewalks or any sort of asphalt, that she needs the feel of the earth under her feet, and this is the umpteenth piece of private property she has tromped across without an ounce of hesitation. In other countries, like Scotland, say, there are right-to-ramble laws promising that no well-intentioned flaneur can be stopped for trespassing. But this is not Scotland, it is the good old US of

A, where fences and walls are considered sacrosanct and the Castle Doctrine is held in high esteem, making property lines the equivalent of invisible moats promising scalding oil and flaming arrows (aka bullets) if crossed. Dot just steps over a row of planted greenery, then barrels across the grass on which a ranch house sits. Meanwhile, I follow on tiptoes, casting nervous, sneaky looks over my shoulder—a sadly reduced version of the adventure-huzzah! author that I initially tried to present myself as for this interview. Dot clocks my unease and assures me, "People don't mind. Why would they mind? I'm enjoying their yard."

Clearly this is a case of white privilege—if either of us were Black or brown there would be no such shenanigans. But this is also a case of homeowner-can't-be-bothered-to-intervene. Let's be honest, a ninety-three-year-old woman in a floppy hat and sensible winter vest doesn't look like trouble. Though Dot does not look or move like a ninety-three-year-old— even standing still she has the nervy excitement of a young baseball player taking his turn at bat. It is only her slight shoulder stoop and her white hair, which flows past high cheekbones and the requisite wrinkles, that might give her away. Now she high-steps beside me, as if walking's normal range of motion isn't energetic enough for her, reminding me of being near a skittish colt—who also happens to know Buddhist texts and quote poetry. Many people in this quiet college town are familiar with Dot Fisher-Smith anyway; they know the woman who bicycled these streets until she was ninety-two. They know the woman who, at eighty-nine, hiked the teeth-gritting, thigh-burning eight-mile-uphill Long Valley trail in the nearby Trinity Alps. They know the woman who spent two nights alone on Mount Shasta just last year, hiking from seventy-eight hundred feet to eighty-two hundred feet and sleeping there. ("I'm happiest at altitude," she tells me.)

This simple propulsion—of one foot leaving the ground, returning to it, then the other leaving the ground—is available to most of us. In the near past, walking was mocked as too gentle, too simple, too downright easy, but these attributes are precisely what makes it a preferred and lauded activity as we age, and it's why I am here today, gamely trying to keep up with Dot. Even younger people have embraced walking as a viable exercise, as the advent of pedometers in our phones and on our watches has made it easy to log how much movement we've managed to squeeze into our mostly sedentary lives. Who hasn't been in the presence of that annoying person who in the late afternoon suddenly, apropos of nothing, announces the number of "steps" accomplished that day? Some people, who will go unnamed, but could possibly be my very own wife, will even offer to walk the dog in my stead in order to get all their steps in, ten thousand being the touted magic number, for reasons that remain a little shady—perhaps because it's a satisfying round number that echoes things like the ten thousand hours of practice the writer Malcolm Gladwell claims will master a skill, or resounds of the divine Ten Commandments, or maybe it actually does take almost five miles of movement in a day to remain fit. In fact, recent studies show that seven thousand to eight thousand daily steps for the middle-aged (about thirty to forty-five minutes of exercise) give the most bang for the buck—more than that doesn't significantly improve your longevity (exercise a lot less than that, though, and your chance of dying young increases 40 percent). The upshot is that walking as exercise has rocketed to popularity. All we need is our two feet, maybe some sneakers or walking shoes, and a safe space through which to ambulate. Sometimes this is on a treadmill in a gym. Sometimes this is at a local high school track. And sometimes, as with Dot, it is up the face of a vertiginous, thin-aired mountain.

When I first told Dot about my own quest to figure out how best to keep adventuring into older age, she'd quickly become indignant. Old? You're not old, she'd exclaimed. "It's ridiculous—pardon my extreme language—it's ridiculous to me that at fifty-seven you could be thinking about how to keep going. Just do what you've always done—it gets better as you get older."

Better? I'd asked her, surprised. And then probed: "Do you mean better emotionally or better physically?" Certainly physically, she answered. "I hiked Ladakh [in the Himalayas] when I was sixty-seven!" she exclaimed. "It's just the beginning. Your best hiking is still to come!"

Later she admits to me that this wisdom had not been easily won. Turning fifty had offered "wonder and amazement"— she'd come so far, done so much, and there was still time to do more—but as her sixtieth birthday approached, she'd fallen into a depression. "I felt like it was the end of the world for me. I felt like, I'm going down the dark side of the mountain." So, in preparation for her imminent demise, she planned a three-day ceremony and invited all the dear people in her life. "I was going to shave my head," she tells me, "and do a death and rebirth ritual." During the run-up to the event she had a conversation with her mother-in-law, who was eighty-six at the time. "She said to me, 'I don't know why you're so upset—the sixties were the best years of my life.' I can hear her voice saying that now. And I've told that to probably fifty people, because the sixties *were* the best years of my life."

But even before that, in her later fifties ("your age," she points out), Dot decided to do what most of us in her solidly middle-class position perhaps can but won't—with the offspring now well out of the house, she and her husband packed up their home, stored or sold their possessions, and headed out for an open-ended ("but at least a year") trip around the world. Nothing about it was upscale—they would be doing it on the savings they had earned as couples counselors—and the focus would be, of course, hiking. Dot wanted to begin with a trek to Everest base camp. They didn't join a group or even hire porters, as almost all tourists do, but instead set off on their own carrying everything they needed themselves. For three months they trekked, stopped at teahouses, trekked. "We were like kids," she says of their bare-bones travel. From there it was on to Burma, then Malaysia, Thailand, New Zealand. "We weren't fancy. We did everything on the cheap."

It would be easy to attribute Dot's astonishing vitality at ninety-three to the simple fact that she has spent so much of her life walking; yes, studies prove over and over that older people who exercise are rewarded with lower blood pressure, increased muscle strength, improved heart health, and a plethora of new brain cells, facilitating learning and memory. But Dot also insists on being outside when she walks, and this, it turns out, may be the more important reason for her crackling energy and ageless pizzazz.

In her book *The Nature Fix*, the author Florence Williams looks at study after study and corroborates what those of us who love being in the wild already know, but can't explain except through incoherent, excitable anecdotes filled with soaring adjectives and dramatic pauses. Williams doesn't bother with the poetics (though she does write beautifully of nature's impact on her) and instead looks at hard biological evidence—traveling to, among other places, Japan, Finland, Norway, and Singapore where extensive studies have proven that nature itself is vital for our health. Williams writes of research so conclusive that the governments of these countries fund parks and forests intentionally built for its citizens to wander through, biologically resting their brain and destressing their hormonal system. In Finland, you might stroll the Power Trail, a path through green space marked intermittently by signposts that guide the perambulator to relax, stretch, and look. In Japan, acres of woods are devoted solely to the practice of *Shinrin-yoku*, or forest bathing, wherein you immerse yourself completely by ditching the phone and other distractions and strolling with all five senses opened to the healing that sloshes among the trees.

Right now, Dot and I are settling for a suburban gambol, though Dot is making it as rural as possible by insisting that we keep our proximity to grass and bushes, ownership be damned. She's onto something: it turns out that chemicals released by trees, called phytoncides, strengthen our immune system and lower blood pressure. Meanwhile, the sounds of rushing wind, whispering leaves, and flowing water measurably relax and focus us, and studies show that birdsong elevates both our mood and our cognitive ability; the sound of happy, preening birds may signal to our primitive selves that no predators are about. (Urban noise, on the other hand, triggers cortisol and blood pressure spikes, and causes the amygdala, the fight-or-flight area of the brain, to go on high alert.) The general prognosis from all these studies is that fifteen to forty-five minutes in a natural setting of any sort increases well-being; five hours a month is the prescription for ongoing emotional and physical restoration. More is better, though, and the wilder and more remote the green space, the better it is for you.

Dot had initially declared that we would be walking to a pond, but after observing the zigzag way we are traveling, I wonder aloud what specific map directions we are following, and Dot admits that she is guided more by sensual waypoints than specific left and right turns. She finds the sun when she wants to be in sun and shade when she wants shade, and of course grass and soil as often as possible. Yes, we are walking to the pond, she tells me, but we are also following the vagaries of destiny. Pomegranates on the tree? Stop to marvel. Leaves turning a vibrant orange? Redirect to look closer.

"If I see something, I stop. If the grass is inviting, I sit down," she says, shrugging. She explains this less as whimsy and more as *beshert*, a Hebrew word that means "destiny," and a guiding principle in her life. On her walks, beshert calls her to follow what the universe is offering, and, though she may not know it consciously, what is being offered is not just the physical health mentioned above, but measurable cognitive rewards, often by calming the activity in our brain. This rest, much like meditation, means increased memory and neural nimbleness once the brain is reengaged. What accounts for this relaxation of the brain? Some studies think that it's the rounded, fractal visual elements of the outdoors matching well with the way our retina is built, allowing for an ease in processing. Nature is also relatively uncluttered; the brain, which is constantly filtering stimuli, is less overworked than in an urban setting, with its racing traffic, sudden loud noises, and hard, linear architecture. All of this results in a lowering of frenetic brain waves in the part of our brain responsible for daily decisions and logistics. Gym-hardened workout fanatics trumpet the importance of rest in order for muscles to build and strengthen, and so it is with the brain. No wonder participants showed significant improvement in memory and cognition after a ramble around green space. No wonder Dot is as sharp as anyone I know, of any age.

Dot is veering onto grass, then stopping suddenly to speak a thought, arms waving for emphasis. Her energy is barely containable. But every now and then she pointedly halts, and I hear her murmur words that, when I ask, turn out to be "Pay attention, practice, relax." She repeats this sentence a few times to herself, then bounds forward again. She explains that with this mantra she is redirecting her sometimes chaotic energy and focus; she is telling herself to slow down. "Right this minute" is also something she will say, she tells me. It puts her firmly back into the present moment, where she feels best—otherwise her energy sags and she feels lost and disconnected.

Soon unseen divine influence hits again and Dot picks up the pace, deciding that walking fast for a while will be good for us. When she stops a few moments later to quote me whole stanzas of a poem by memory, it's easy to see birdsong, phytoncides, and languid theta waves at work. This, despite the fact that Dot did not grow up in the outdoors. Her parents, she tells me, "would never walk anywhere that they could drive to." Her childhood was spent in the segregated South, and Dot hated it, from a young age knowing that the racism and hierarchies she saw all around her were wrong. She lived in a succession of apartments, far from green spaces, and "never knew where anything came from." Butter, fruit—it never occurred to her that these things had a beginning elsewhere, and a journey before arriving on her plate. Her parents lived an indoor life, their true passion the game of bridge (her mother was the first woman to be a Life Master in the American Contract Bridge League), and Dot remembers with disdain their days and nights of smoking and drinking and cards. She vowed not to be like them ("I never learned to play bridge. I've never smoked a cigarette in my life. And I never drive anywhere I can walk"). Finally, in her teens, she left the South during the summers ("escaped," she tells me) and stayed with family friends who had a second home in Woodstock, New York. There, she swam in creeks and "met real people," including Hans, the young man Dot describes as her "first true love." His mother was the "original hippie," Dot tells me, someone who wore dirndls and had long gray hair and drove a Model T Ford; he was recently home from World War II, where he had been guarding bridges in China. All this allowed her to see a life outside of the bigotry, the bridge-playing, the car-driving, the smoking and drinking, of her parents. Something was germinating, something that would be an integral part of the rest of her life, but she couldn't see it yet. Upon graduating from high school, she attended Tulane, but left after a year for upstate New York and Hans. It became a pivotal time, when she shed old notions of herself as an outsider who had never had boyfriends, "a self-conscious Jewish girl." Partly this was the glow of newfound love (she and Hans moved in together—"It was called 'living in sin' back then," she tells me wryly—and eventually married), but partly something else happened: Hans took her hiking in the

Green Mountains. "Suddenly, I knew why I was alive," she says now. Dot had found love, she had found nature, and she had found walking in nature.

I knew why I was alive. "It was that revelatory?" I asked. How?

"I just told you. Because it's the EARTH," she responds, indignant. *Come on, it's so obvious,* her tone says. Well, yes, it makes sense to me, someone who has been exposed to the outdoors since childhood, but it won't to everyone. For many Americans, a need to maintain contact with the grass and soil sounds a little wacky. Surely a well-laid concrete walkway, or better yet a plush rug, are preferable. Yet scientists and psychologists have seen time and again what Dot knows intuitively, impatiently—the less urban the environment you stroll in, the more well-being you feel. It's good to walk in a city park, but a city park is not as potent as uninterrupted green space farther from our cities and suburbs.

I wait for Dot to continue, but instead she talks of her dread of climate chaos, her anger at the corporations that won't stop their violations of the planet, her sadness at yet another housing development built in her town. Perhaps what she is saying is that you might not yet love the outdoors, you might not even like it much, but be aware that now is your chance, your only chance, to embrace this potent remedy before it is gone.

"It's very painful, every piece of earth that I see covered over. I see the weeds coming up between the cracks of the asphalt and that's telling me: Earth doesn't like it, she's being smothered, she wants to be free." She pauses to stare at me. "Is that clear enough for you?"

The sidewalks are behind us now. We tromp across a field, not somebody's property but city land this time. Dot points ahead—a BMX bike course forms a necklace around a dirt mound. A footbridge rises nearby. And there, a tree where a heron once had a nest. Soon we approach blackened foliage, and Dot tells me this is the ignition point (along with a human hand and a lighter) of the rapacious Almeda wildfire that scorched four thousand acres, swallowed up twenty-eight hundred homes, and killed three people within twenty-four hours. We are a little quieter for a few moments after that, pondering the enormity of that disaster and all the pending future ones that climate change will bring. The disappearance of nature is real, and will exert its own deadly pall both on our emotional and on our physical selves. When over a hundred million trees died through an insect infestation of the emerald ash borer, there was a correlating increase in cardiovascular and respiratory human deaths in the area. A shocking fifteen thousand more people died of heart problems. Six thousand more over the norm died of respiratory illnesses. Trees are filters, inhalers of polluting CO_2, givers of oxygen, regulators of air temperature. On the most basic, physiological level—breath itself—trees are life-giving for us.

Then Dot simply says, "The pond." And there it is before us: small, dark-watered, the littoral bushes adding a shaggy feel. Despite its lack of pomposity, or majesty, or Dot's warning from the beginning that it wouldn't compare to the alpine lakes she most adores, I nevertheless feel the soothing effects of water and trees right away. Ducks glide by. The sun comes out from behind the clouds. As we come upon a bench, I ask Dot to sit on it with me for a minute. I am intrigued by benches, I explain. They are an offering from some anonymous human. *Sit, look, here's a view and I want you to see it.*

Dot likes to move, seems compelled to do so, but when I say, "A bench is a moment to sit on," she ponders this statement, repeats it, then nods her approval and sits. Dot has many great qualities, and right now I see yet another one: she is open to a new experience, even one as quotidian as bench sitting. Dot's sixties may have been her favorite decade, but her hiking did not slow even as she passed seventy. At seventy-three she completed, with a friend, the month-long trek from Leh to Manali in the Himalayas. At seventy-five, she and John (who was seventy-seven) traveled to Tibet and trekked the sacred Kora trail, which circles the holiest mountain in Asia, Mount Kailash. The walk, which they did with four other friends, is stratospherically arduous.

"You are crossing the high plateau for weeks to get there," she tells me. "It's a *biiig* trip. And we did it. John almost didn't make it—the pass that you cross is at 18,500."

"Why did you want to do it?" I ask.

"Why would I NOT want to do it?" she shoots back, disgusted with me again. How could I even ask? Then she lists the reasons. "Because it's the sacred mountain. Because I love the Himalayas. Because I was a Soto Zen practitioner for thirty-five years. And I love hiking."

We don't dally long on the bench. As I said, Dot's natural state is movement, which is why I was nervous to go on this walk to begin with. When I'd proposed that we meet, Dot had excitedly offered a saunter up Grizzly Peak. Just the words "Grizzly," which I'd interpreted as Grisly, and "Peak" made me hesitate, to which she had exclaimed, "It's totally tame! It's just a five-mile hike!" Reluctantly, I admitted that I had, um, limitations. Could we do a gentle walk instead? Three miles, max? Dot duly softened and asked me to explain.

I dislike discussing my injuries—especially to someone thirty-five years older than I. But I present as fit and robust, so most of the time they do need explaining. I spell out my situation: a fall in a fire as a San Francisco firefighter led to many surgeries and finally one replaced knee at the relatively tender age of forty-one. More of consequence is the remade ankle, full of metal and cadaver bone from a bad landing (also known as a "crash") in an ultralight aircraft, which I, an experienced pilot, was flying.

But really, what active person arrives at my age without aches and pains? Dot, apparently. Her first real injury came at age ninety. That was when she tripped while roughhousing with a dog and broke her femur. Within a week she was out of the hospital (amazing) and doing rehab at her home. Indeed, I could not have guessed from her speedy and balanced gait today that a mere three years ago she had broken the biggest bone in her body. More recently, at ninety-two, she was trying out a new bike and lost her balance as she was getting the hang of it. The pedal took a chunk out of her calf, which became infected. This resulted in a nine-month saga of rest, reinfection, rest again. Both of those incidences were "a huge teaching for me," she muses, and she assures me that they enable her to have (some) sympathy for my gimpy state (before that, she admits, other people's frailty—breaking bones, lying in hospital beds—was not even on her radar).

We leave the pond behind and traverse the city's scorched field once more. Then, back among the sidewalks and houses, set off again "cross country," as Dot calls it. As we near her residence, she expresses dismay at her current living situation, in a senior facility just blocks from her old house (John is in the assisted-care wing of the same place). "I'm an ageist. I don't like old people. I didn't consider myself old, even when I was old."

Indeed, she shows me around her studio apartment as if it were a temporary living space, though she has made it undeniably welcoming and cozy. It spills over with notebooks and talismans from her travels. On the walls hangs her art: numinous collages made with sticks and poetry, beautifully rendered mountain ranges painted on weathered canvas. The canvas was cut from an old meditation yurt, Dot tells me, that had to be scrapped when it was ripped up by curious cows. Lichen-spotted, sun-bleached, rain-stained, it offered shapes and forms that she then allowed "the pen, graphite, colored pencils, and pastels to tease out." And it wasn't just the old canvas that was given new life: all the materials she used were secondhand ("I'm a recycler," she says), including a boxed set of French portrait pastels inherited from John's grandfather. But despite this pageantry of art and amulets, the small footprint of the room makes it hard to avoid a carceral feel, and Dot's restless energy confirms that this is not where she wants to be, she has other plans for her future.

. . .

I forget to check the steps recorded on my phone during our walk, remembering only after they are muddled with subsequent dog ambles and gym routines. Not that Dot cares—she has no use for petty measurements (when I'd mentioned step counters before our walk, she'd looked at me with a little pity). Instead, Dot understands walking's essential gifts, and they are all non-metric—physical movement, scintillating discussions, nature. A power amble up the side of a mountain would have been more her style, yes. When I'd mentioned on the phone that I would be happy to just hang out in a prone position on my paddleboard as long as I was on a beautiful waterway with wildlife all around me, she'd offered up, first, a long pause, and then a slightly harrumph-y "Oh, no. No. I could never just sit there." For Dot, this walk was a mere jaunt, a languid shuffle. Was this still beneficial?

Exercise presumes some set amount of time (usually a minimum of thirty minutes) and a particular amount of exertion (monitored by heart rate or, more colloquially, by how easily you can speak at the same time). Undeniably, it's good for us. Less well known are the new studies that tout mere movement as a health requirement. Pace while you talk on the telephone instead of sitting in a chair. Put clean laundry in its drawers in multiple trips instead of efficiently, all at one time. Take the stairs instead of the elevator: at Dot's residential complex there was always someone standing outside the elevator, peering at the numbers impatiently, but Dot never once gave it a glance, making a beeline to the stairwell each time, to and from her apartment on the fourth floor. This kind of random, constant movement puts us in touch with our biological selves, and offers meaningful benefits. For those who need numbers: an overview of seventy-two studies showed that glucose and insulin levels drop with "short but frequent bouts of light-intensity activity compared with continuous sitting." Surprisingly, it may also help cardiovascular health. Overall, there is a strong suggestion from the data that you will simply live longer if you move more.

My outing with Dot was mostly just that, *movement*. But we had been awash in nature, which is such a potent elixir. And Dot's ability to be delighted by little things—the soil, the grass, the trees, our conversation—added an exhilaration

I hadn't expected. Exhilaration, I was beginning to see, doesn't need adrenaline. It can be triggered by that simple act of paying attention.

There was also the undeniable psychological hurdle I had just stepped over. I have battled pain in my ankle and knees for years. But today I had participated in, not quite a hike, not really even a walk, more a stop-and-start peregrination. But I felt *good*. I might ice when I get home, or I might not need to. No, really, I felt pretty great. This was undergirded by the grass under my sneakers, the proximity to leaves, soil, and water, and, last but not least, the joy of communing with a remarkable human being. I would give walking (or random peregrination) greater attention now, add it to my list of future outdoor activities. Maybe I'd keep it to "movement" or maybe I'd amp up the pace, to make it exercise. Either way it was a win.

While in her apartment, Dot flipped through journals of past hikes. They told of high passes, soaring views, good weather and bad. She said she was planning her next excursion (which a few months later would become a reality: twenty-seven hundred feet of elevation gain, seven miles, three days, a twenty-pound pack). Then she read me a haiku she had written.

> When I go outside
> Every tree and blade of grass
> Tells me I'm alive.

5

Adapt

We all have issues. The secret to successful aging is to recognize one's issues and adapt accordingly.

—JANE BRODY, AGE EIGHTY, FORMER *NEW YORK TIMES* HEALTH COLUMNIST

Here is the strange and mystical language spoken this morning:

"Who cooks for you? Who cooks for you?" asks a woman to my left in a low chant.

"Teakettle teakettle," quietly answers another perfectly sane human.

"Quick pick up the beer check," whispers someone else, though there is not a beer in sight.

"Sweet Canada, sweet Canada," another suddenly interrupts.

It could be a gathering of lullaby writers. Or perhaps a strange game of charades. Instead, the people around me are birdwatchers, and we are in a park in Austin, Texas, where the sun hasn't even risen, and we are mere looming, lurking shadows on a mazy path among trees. But the air is trilling and these humans around me are not losing their minds; instead they are identifying the song of certain birds in the vicinity. We are here for what is called the Dawn Chorus, that time around sunrise where birds begin to announce themselves and their randy, territorial intentions before the full day begins. The weed whackers and leaf blowers are still silent, the temperature cool, the insects not yet visible enough for feeding to be in order. Instead all around we are being treated to this soft acoustic set, akin to some waifish twenty-something singing onstage, nothing operatic, not earthshaking, but stirring nevertheless.

This is the first of many surprises about birdwatching—that bird-watching is actually also bird-*listening*. It is also bird-imitating, bird-speculating, bird-dreaming.

Great-tailed grackle! Nashville warbler! Mourning dove!

I am here because birding seems like an outdoor activity that accommodates our inevitable physical slowing as we age. Through birding, I thought, outdoor adventure might remain within reach for almost all of us. But what do I know, I haven't really birded before, so who better to help me explore this theory than Virginia Rose, age sixty-four, who now pulls up alongside me in her wheelchair. Virginia is Caucasian, slight of build, with enviable cheekbones and shoulder-length gray hair topped by a ball cap. Her no-nonsense efficiency combined with her good looks and cheer remind me of a flight attendant, but she also can't quite contain her energy—she wouldn't hand you peanuts so much as throw them at you with a grin and move on. Every time I glance her way she is smiling, and it's not for show. It seems to be her natural state: sparkling eyes, small half smile, an air of listening.

"Hear that chip?" she asks me now. "It has a *pink* to it, a metallic sound." I nod and cock my head, staring toward the dark hummocks of flora, blinking to try to bring something into focus. But eyes don't do much right now, and instead into my brain seeps whirs and clicks and peeps I hadn't initially perceived; to my surprise, I *do* hear it. Virginia watches my face closely, lit as it is a ghostly green by the pathway lighting. Smiling, she tracks my expression as I register the call. "Northern cardinal," she says, and I feel suddenly a small connection to the wild world, that little fizz of joy at something that has slipped into place, even as I didn't realize anything was out of place to begin with.

There are nine of us out here this morning, some in wheelchairs, some "walking people," as Virginia likes to say. This is the beginning of a "birdathon" where we will visit six parks in the next twelve hours, logging birds as we go (and covering a whopping six and a half miles); the information will then be sent through an app to ongoing ornithology studies. All around the country birders are participating in this seasonal citizen science, which documents how spring migratory paths may be changing, which species are thriving, and which species are not.

Titmouse! Crow! Cooper's!

The walking people consist of Celeste, fifty-seven, a veterinarian who likes to throw out puns; Jeff, sixty, a quiet bear of a man described to me as the most knowledgeable birder of the group, who demurs on this; Connie, age sixty-four, who attends Virginia's book club; and Kira, a young woman of thirty new to birding but getting good at picking out birds, mostly visually, she tells me, as the calls and songs still stump her. Kira has learned because for the past year she has worked as the caregiver to Eric, thirty-four, who uses a motorized wheelchair, and who, it quickly becomes clear, has a gift for hearing and identifying birdsong, a technique called ear-birding. Also with us is Kathey, sixty-eight, a longtime birder who has used a wheelchair for seven years and "birded" throughout. "You can do everything in a wheelchair," she tells me, almost fiercely. "It's just a lot harder." And of course, there is Virginia, our fearless leader, the organizer of today's birdathon.

. . .

The marathon quality of this venture certainly runs counter to birding's reputation as a sedate hobby, executed at a slow amble or from the comfort of a porch. This is yet another truth about birding that surprises: yes, there is speaking in hushed tones, yes, there is slow forward movement, yes, there are long periods of silence, but to confuse that with sedateness would be foolish. These are just the tools of the trade that allow for birds to appear. There are indeed "bird sits," where one parks oneself in one place and watches what birds come around. But there are also "bird brawls," where an intrepid birder tries to cover lots of ground to log more birds than an opponent. There are also the informal ambles you take on your own—Virginia may be a social creature, but she also loves to bird without other people, she tells me. As different as each of these birding avenues are, they all seem to be done with the same ebullience and passion.

As the sky lightens, the park itself begins to take shape—wide path, pretty meadow, and up ahead, a pond. Bird movement is now added to our spotting technique: barn swallows doing their jerky breakdance, the glint of disturbed leaves that hints at a chickadee. Virginia pushes forward in her manual wheelchair and comments on the terrain of crushed gravel—"It's a walking person's vision of accessible," she tells me. She points out what I would otherwise have missed—it's not well packed, there's a slight incline, and with so much crunching and pinging under-wheel, it can be hard to hear the birds.

Virginia has been in a wheelchair since a fall from a horse at fourteen. She says her parents hardly treated her differently after that, and were firm in their belief that Virginia and her two walking sisters could do anything they set their mind to. "We were taught by our parents that there is never a day in your life to be bored. There's so much to do, it was just all about being curious, then go out and figure out what was interesting all around you. They never told me, 'So sorry you're in a wheelchair.'"

Virginia didn't find birding until midlife. Until then she had been doing what many people in their twenties and thirties do—barhopping, concerts, and "being in places you want to be seen." At forty-two, "I was done with all that, and I thought, What's the next thing?" She was trying to figure out how to spend a Friday night when she came across a lecture at the local Audubon Society, on house finches. *House finches?* scoffed her friends, wondering how a tiny local bird could appeal to a firecracker like Virginia. "I told them, I don't know. But I went. Immediately I was enthralled. It was an instant attraction. I was that obnoxious person asking all the questions." (This makes the house finch her "spark bird," that particular winged creature that triggers one's birding passion.) After the lecture Virginia wheeled back to her car and phoned her mother. "I asked her, 'Why didn't you tell me I was such a nerd? Life would have been so much easier.'"

She was still a high school English teacher but would bird as often as possible. "Oh, my gosh, birding can fill an entire life, learning all the birds, learning all the songs, all the bird habitat, educating yourself on the mannerisms. It's nonstop. You'll never get it all done. I love that. Nature, in such a unique way, offers that kind of lifelong purpose."

For years Virginia birded on her own or with walking people. It brought her back into relationship with the outdoors in ways she had not felt since she was a child. With that came confidence, stamina and strength from wheeling to and fro, and that sense of purpose. It also brought with it epiphanies. "Walking people would always venture off on their own where I couldn't go. Once I was by myself, listening so acutely to the sounds, watching the sunlight and the shadows and the leaves and the wind blowing. And all of a sudden, I was overcome. I realized in that moment I was looking at my best self, and I was the happiest I've ever been. It was very visceral. I felt I was delivered." Another insight came soon after: Why didn't she ever see anybody else birding in a wheelchair? Like a true evangelist she decided it must simply be because they hadn't heard about bird-watching, so she set about spreading the good word. She gave presentations at the local spinal-cord-injury meeting, at the amputee support group, at multiple sclerosis and stroke support groups. She spoke to rehabilitation therapists. She posted information in the rehab gyms and on the walls of hospitals. Virginia believed that just getting outside would be empowering, of course. But doing it while connecting with birds—that would be mind-blowing and life-changing. *Come birding!* was her essential message, *come birding!,* an incantation like a dawn song.

When I ask why birding is such a palliative, other birders have answers. Celeste tells me that the outdoors is vital, sure ("a bad day birding is still a good day," she says), but birding adds that extra element of novelty. "You're always learning something," she tells me. Terry, who joins us at the second park and stays for the rest of the day, is a walking person and a retired labor and delivery nurse, who explains, "It's the pleasure of *Ah, I found one.* It's like an Easter egg hunt."

For Eric, birding offers something else. He explains later in an email that he began to use a wheelchair at eighteen, as his particular form of muscular dystrophy progressed. "For much of my life, I've shied away from adventure, but through birding, I've been able to reconnect with other parts of myself: bravery, resilience, a willingness to take on new risks." I love hearing this, because for many people "birding" and "adventure" aren't something they expect in the same sentence. "Birding inspires me to step outside my comfort zone in a way that no other activities do," he says. And now, with only a few hours and two parks under my birding belt, I can see what he is talking about: the experience has already been marked by adrenaline spikes, thumps of joy, stretches of boredom, and waves of exhilaration—in sum, it has its own sort of intensity and all the hallmarks of outdoor adventure.

Virginia agrees with all of this. "I'm excited as a kid at Christmas when I finally see a bird that I've been listening to for half an hour." But she mostly loves the way birding guides one to pay attention. "Birding is a way to be present. It means you're absorbed in the Right Now. The whole purpose is to listen closely, to watch closely, to be aware of movement and time and season and habitat and all of the things that make up being in the present—I think I just heard a blue-gray gnat-catcher. Nobody goes to museums with me, because I read every placard and stare at every painting. The same is true of birding—redwing blackbird, that tree." She cocks her head away and then back at me. "That's psychology 101 for an anxious moment, right?—ruby-crowned kinglet—feel your hands, watch your breathing. That's birding."

It's ironic that Virginia is talking about being in the moment while multitasking birds. Isn't that the epitome of fractured attention? But then I am reminded of a story I heard in a college class on Buddhism. In it, a monk tumbles off a cliff. On the way down to his certain death, filled with all the attendant emotions of surprise and regret and fear, he manages to catch sight of a beautiful strawberry growing from the rock face, and he plucks it as he tumbles past. As a twenty-year-old, I had no idea what this story was supposed to teach. Did this hapless monk love fruit so much? Did death not matter in the face of a passing berry? No, the professor said. This is about the ability to be in the moment, even as the moment rushes you toward your certain demise. It is about being so attuned to the present that you can spot and then appreciate a tiny strawberry even as you hurtle by it at great speed with other things on your mind. In a similar manner, birders can hold a conversation with you, but they are also always seeing and hearing the strawberry, as long as that straw-berry is a flycatcher or a wren. Therefore, what Virginia says is manifestly true in the deeply Buddhist sense: birding teaches you to pay attention.

Virginia eventually founded Birdability, which strives to connect birding to people with access challenges. The group leads birding outings (today's birdathon is a Birdability event), but Virginia understood early that information on parks lacked vital details for those with disabilities. So she drew up a list of factors that would be of concern: slope, accessible bathrooms, path construction, and railing heights (note to walking people: many railings obstruct the sight line of a person in a wheelchair). When she spoke at a National Audubon Society convention in 2019 about this, Audubon members took the idea and ran with it, eventually creating crowdsourced facts on parks all around the country. The "Birdability maps," as they are called on the Birdability website, answered a set of questions that began with Virginia's list—is the bathroom sink low enough for someone in a wheelchair? How steep are the trails?—but expanded to take into account more disabilities, something that surprised and delighted Virginia. There were so many limitations beyond mobility that she hadn't considered. Would a blind person, required to ear-bird, find a park near an airport untenable? What are the needs of someone on the autism spectrum? Would a person with hearing issues want to avoid birding before the sun comes up, when there is no light, just the dawn song with which to distinguish birds?

The first Birdability outing included a person with COPD, a respiratory disease—"This is why benches are so important," Virginia tells me; another who was obese and used a scooter; someone else with MS in a motorized chair. The birding was of interest, but soon enough the group, all of whom were strangers, began to chatter among themselves. "They were looking at each other and comparing caster wheels, backpacks, shoes. That's when it dawned on me." Birding, she realized, was precious access to the outdoors, and to birds. But it was also access to community.

Birding is also accessible in other ways—economically. Besides the time input (a precious resource), it is inexpensive. Even binoculars are not required, as so many birders do much of their birding through listening. Eric, who does not have the ability to hold binoculars himself, is by necessity an ear-birder, and only asks Kira once or twice if he can look through her binoculars during our excursion.

One cannot think birding and inclusiveness, though, without remembering the white woman who called the police on Christian Cooper, a Black bird-watcher in Central Park, after Cooper asked the woman to leash her dog per park rules, so the birds wouldn't be disturbed. Luckily, there is a proliferation of Black birders, as well as organizations for birdy people of color that offer formal outings and, with that, relative safety.

"What's that twittering?" Celeste asks Jeff. "Chimney swift," he answers. There is a brief aside about how the wrens fly—"Zip! Zip!" Virginia mimics, nodding. (Later, when she reenacts the way a bird eats, by shaking her head back and forth to smash a phantom caterpillar against a phantom branch with a phantom beak, she laughingly tells me: "Birders have no shame!")

Nashville warbler! Red-bellied woodpecker!

Many birders compile ongoing life lists, composed of all the species they've seen, with their sights set on species they want to see (a "lifer") and indeed today we are listing, too, in this case for science. (In the end we will spot fifty-two separate species.) Virginia keeps a list for herself, but it isn't a priority. "Most people can tell you how many different birds they've seen in their life. But I can't. I get a little fussy about that. I think, Please, don't make me beholden to any mark or procedure." Celeste agrees. "I'm a Type A personality to begin with, and birding is a mindfulness practice for me. I've intentionally not become a lister—scissortail!" The group responds with exhales of appreciation. Indeed, the scissor-tailed flycatcher is an especially stunning bird, with its salmon-colored belly, gray head, and absurdly long two-bladed tail.

It isn't just bird lists. Virginia tells me she was assisting in a divorce recovery class that asked its participants to write down ten things that made them happy. She decided to play along and quickly had a list, too—fifty items long. "Find all the art galleries, visit one a week. Find all the city parks, visit one a week. Find all the museums, the little theaters," she remembers. "How to live your best life is to make sure you're exploring."

Kira turns to a sound. I ask what it is. "Cardinal," she says, pointing to a bright red bird. When I gasp with appreciation, she smiles. "Everyone loves the cardinal," she tells me. It's common to the area, she adds, but that doesn't take away from its beauty.

We are at our third park, circling a new pond, and suddenly Jeff says, "Green heron." No one sees it yet, but evidently it has called. I've never even known there was such a bird as a green heron, let alone heard its cry.

Calls, I come to learn, differ from songs. Celeste explains patiently that songs are used to declare territory and attract mates, they are unique to each species, and mostly it's the males that sing, though some species have singing females, too. Calls, on the other hand, are generic chips, fusses, and alarms—short repetitive sounds all birds use, mostly to chat— *Hey, how are you, when are you coming home with the groceries*—or to alert others that a predator is about. Birders identify birds through calls as well as song, because each species' sounds are tonally and rhythmically different. Now, Celeste cups a hand behind each ear and says, "That. That's wet sounding. Do you hear it? A *seep* versus a *zeep*, which is more like a zipper." I don't hear it, but I appreciate the nuance and the way she is practicing a deep listening that I'm coming to admire, and even to emulate.

Birders consider many things during bird identification: habitat (that it's Austin, Texas, but also is the bird in a tree or on the ground?), what time of year (the clay-colored sparrow won't be seen in summer), the shape (of the beak, of the wings), structure (how steep is the forehead, is the body elongated), feathers, color, song, call. All this engages the birder in a mystery of sorts, full of deductive reasoning, and sometimes speculation, that Easter egg hunt that Terry mentioned. But how to begin? The birders seem to shrug at this and say in various ways, *Just begin.* I wonder out loud at how impossible it seems to link birds to all these attributes; perhaps I would never be a real birder. Celeste assures me, "If you're paying attention to birds, then you're birding." Eric agrees, later urging me not to get caught up in the identification at all. "If a wild bird can make you feel alive and present, that's something to cherish." Identification is important, he tells me, "but it should never impede that sense of wonder."

Finally, the green heron makes itself known, sliding across the water. It's not green in the traditional way, but iridescent in the way of a very dark pearl, and it catches my breath. If I hadn't already fallen in love years ago with pelicans, which I watch while surfing, I would claim this bird to be my spark bird, so much does it move me in that moment. Later I look it up on the internet and am slightly disappointed by how drab it looks in its photograph, but that disappointment is tempered when I remember the thrill I felt, how my stomach dropped in the way of new love. I realize that staring at a photo on a screen just can't compare. Nor does it adequately reenact the living, breathing company of the humans I was with, all who had that rare identifying trait of wanting to be amazed, over and over, by each winged creature, so that I too was swept away.

Clay-colored sparrow! American pipit!

Virginia shows me the migration path of the clay-colored sparrow on a map on her phone. "The birds we see here, people are soon going to see in Canada. Isn't that neat?" Indeed it is, giving me a sense of a more connected planet, one not divided by national boundaries but fluid with flyways and air currents, where its creatures are traveling, seeking, thriving, indifferent to your color or status, focused instead on good marshes and fine weather. To bird is not just to notice a creature by the size of its head, the splay of its feathers, or the curve of the beak but to marvel at where it has come from and where it is going, and the fortitude it takes for the journey. Jeff talks about a time he watched a "fallout," where birds coming across a large body of water against a particularly tough headwind plummet exhausted onto land. These are the lucky ones; many are lost at sea if the weather isn't favorable and land isn't near. It was a spectacular way to see a bird migration, Jeff remembers, this giant curtain of live feathers and bodies literally *falling* to the ground to recuperate. "Good for birders," says Terry, "bad for birds." I get another glimpse of just how resonant, then, birds are to humans, with not just plumage and song on display, but sheer will and dogged courage. One can only be awestruck by this long, arduous annual voyage, thousands of miles and back again, a small slice of which I am now lucky enough to witness.

Ladder-backed woodpecker! White-eyed vireo! Purple martin!

Virginia has coined a phrase that goes like this: "Unearth your inner explorer; she is probably your Best Self." But women have a hard time doing that, she tells me, because they don't like venturing outdoors alone. It's not about their safety, she says when I ask. "They just don't—sorry, there, eastern bluebird—don't know how to be alone." They don't know what to *do* with themselves, she explains. "Do not think your greatest accomplishments are going to happen in your comfort zone," she then gently admonishes no one in particular.

Her tough love is right on, but birding itself doesn't require one to be alone and can actually be a gentle way to move outside one's box, because it is an adventure that can be learned in baby steps. Eric tells me he began birding from his window three years earlier after reading Jenny Odell's book *How to Do Nothing*. An avid birder, Odell writes that birding teaches us to pay attention in an otherwise frenetic world, thus connecting us more fully to our surroundings and ourselves. Eric decided to give it a try. As he became more and more attuned to birds in his backyard, he installed a feeder, bringing them in earnest. Soon he was heading to parks and trails. "Birding brought me back to humans," he tells me now.

We're now at our fourth park, and Virginia hasn't slowed down, even though she mentions once that her shoulders are starting to hurt. She doesn't ask for help—there isn't even a proper handle on her wheelchair for a walking person to push. Eventually she asks Eric if she can hitch a ride with him, and he agrees—she holds on to his armrest while he motors them along (she has already broached the etiquette of this to him, and he has told her that it's okay as long as she's careful not to tip over his chair). We stare at a woodpecker hole for a while.

I ask about birding etiquette in general, and Virginia says, "I often have to remind people to look up. But the walking persons don't need that as much as those of us in wheelchairs." Celeste says that if someone mimes bringing binoculars to their eyes, that means everyone should be quiet, something has been spotted. If you want to talk, fall back from the group and use your "birding voice," adds Terry. Terry tells me she dislikes too much talk—you miss the birds, she says, but Virginia shakes her head, laughing, and breaks in, "Birding is about people, too."

The big sighting of the day happens here—the Swainson's hawk. Its finely etched markings stand out against the blue sky. We *ooh* and *ahh* in low voices, the birder version of watching a firework display. Terry finds its call on an app on her phone and we gather around, listening to how it differs from that of a red-tail. "Huskier," says Terry of one of the sounds. "More clipped," says Jeff. (It sounds all the same to me.) Birding can get as nerdy as you want it to be, Jeff tells me, with people hunched over spectrograms to examine the audio waves of a tiny *chip*. For those of us already apprehensive of how technology separates us (and our kids and grandkids) from the outdoors, this might set off our own alarm call, but rest assured that, despite the plethora of technology, the actual birds around us remain the central focus, at least with the birders I'm with. No one buries their faces in their phones, more enamored with the screen version; there is always a strong and unwavering connection to the real-life habitat all around us.

The final park is less accessible, with a steep and rutted downhill path. Virginia decides to descend backward, with Jeff as a spotter. Once we arrive at the bottom, the park redeems itself with a smooth, wide trail and a shelf of limestone, over which water pours into a lazy river. We meander along a meadow of grass and cypress, through which sunlight dapples the ground. We take the time to ponder a milkweed, watch a bee, gawp at the bluebells. For some, a love of the outdoors leads them to birds, but for others it's the opposite. Jeff remarks that for him, "Birding is a gateway drug" to peering more closely at tree species and insects and flowers.

It's nearing sunset, and we are all tired, walking people and those in wheelchairs alike, so we call it a day. Not that birders ever actually stop birding. ("The shift in attention is like a light switch," Eric says. "Only once you begin to notice birds, the switch never turns off.")

As we head back to the parking lot I am reminded of something I read in an article about Virginia. "We are all temporarily able-bodied," she told a birding organization, referring to the fact that even if you are lucky enough to never injure yourself, there is still the inevitable slowing that comes for all of us with age. In fact, I am here today to see how bird-watching accommodates those physical limitations and allows access to an outdoor adventure. But what I find instead is that the gifts are more than that—that bird-watching allows access to the terrain of the present moment and a mindset of complete absorption, free of negative messaging, internal back talk, judgment. It is just all about the bird. And birds are available wherever your particular body needs to be: your window, your stoop, a nearby park. You can bird sit, brawl, or -athon. Virginia stops wheeling, cants her head. "To-woo," she says. "Hear that?" Nodding all around. "With a little flare behind it," Terry adds. "Lesser goldfinch," someone else says. We start up again, that slow birder amble toward our cars, looking like we have somewhere to go, but listening, looking, hoping, just one of many species along an endless flyway.

6

Cultivate Awe

It's just so sad when people say, oh, I'm fifty,
I can't . . . fill in the blank.
Try it anyway! Who cares! You might be surprised.

—DIEDRE WOLOWNICK, WHO BEGAN CLIMBING IN HER
SIXTIES AND SUMMITED EL CAPITAN AT AGE SEVENTY

One day I receive a video: In it a red biplane takes off from a grass field. In the back seat is a man wearing goggles and a flying cap. In the front seat sits a diminutive gray-haired white woman. The picture isn't close-up or all that clear—it's from a wide-angle camera attached to the wing—but she appears to be in her sixties (seventy-one, it turns out) and she could have been piloting, except that as the plane rolls down the runway, she lifts both arms and spreads them to each side (later she told me she was checking to see how a sixty-mile-per-hour wind felt against her hand, for reasons that will soon become clear). The plane rises up over the ocean, and I settle in to watch yet another internet favorite, a picturesque ride in an old-timey plane over beautiful coastline.

Suddenly the camera angle changes. We are looking forward, from the tail. The effect is of being in the plane along with its occupants, with the horizon ahead and your own hair tangling in your eyes. But then a strange thing happens. The woman raises a hand to the wing above her, and feels around. After a few seconds, she seems satisfied she has found what she is looking for (a handle, it turns out). Another hand drifts upward, finds a hold. Then, holy cow, the woman stands. Swiftly, she puts a foot on the side of the plane and pushes. Suddenly it is clear what she is doing. She is getting up on the wing. From my place in the back of the plane—no, wait, actually, I'm in the comfort of my desk chair, peering at my computer screen—I reflexively gasp *"What!?"* and grip my knees.

The next few minutes of the video feature the woman grinning madly from the top of the biplane, where she has attached herself with some sort of harness to a king post. The horizon suddenly dips, then spins behind her; the pilot is executing a series of dastardly loops and rolls. At one point the woman raises her arm and appears to shout.

Later Cynthia Hicks, now seventy-three, tells me she was shouting, "Thank you, God, for keeping my cancer away! Thank you, God, for letting me be here today!"

I reach Cynthia on the telephone through her daughter, who had posted the video on the internet and titled it "Mamma went Wing Walking!!" (Underneath it continued, ". . . without a word about it to us kids. Maybe one day she will learn to act her age . . . nah!") I had some burning questions for this woman who had set her sights on this bizarre outdoor endeavor and mastered it.

My first question for Cynthia was the one we all might ask: WHY? Surely wing walking is for the young and dumb. It is for those seeking their next Instagram moment, or for drunken bragging rights to impress a date.

"I just keep looking for another challenge," Cynthia tells me. She says this without irony, even as I am enumerating in my head many other challenging options like, say, learning a language, or mastering French cooking. She adds, "When I go to a new place I google 'Something Fun to Do Here.'"

"Something Fun to Do Here" eventually turned up wing walking.

She explains that she watched the ensuing videos on the internet with interest. People clambering around on a biplane with their faces distended by the wind, arms skyward in a Rocky pose once they had harnessed themselves to the center post—it all looked pretty appealing to her, actually. (Not surprisingly, she had already tried bungee jumping.) She was sure she had the guts to do it, but was it something that she could do physically? Cancer just seven years before, at sixty-four, had been arduous. "That was a whole year of getting my breast removed, chemo, and radiation." Then it was another year of working out in the gym to get back into shape. At the time she only planned six months in advance, because she had a 50 percent chance of being alive in five years.

Cynthia passed the five-year mark and was now officially in remission. Hallelujah! Here was a second chance at life. What, then, did friends and family say when Cynthia told them of her wing walking plans? Her decision might have seemed much like that of a gambler who wins big, then decides to stay at the table and keep playing. "Oh, I didn't tell anyone," Cynthia tells me. "In case I chickened out."

Wing walking, which began in the 1920s as one of the many ways to wow crowds at "barnstorming" airshows, is defined as any movement across the wing of a flying plane. Today, it isn't really a thing; most people think I've mumbled "woodworking," or said "ring walking," perhaps a strange Druid custom. But back then it was all the rage, and often featured tricks like transferring from a moving car to a low-flying plane wing, or hopping from one aircraft to another in midair, or even hanging from one's teeth. It was not uncommon for pilots to crash performing increasingly outrageous feats, like flying through an actual barn, so by 1927 low-level aerobatics were banned, and barnstorming faded, and with it, wing walking. Mason Wing Walking Academy, in Sequim, Washington, is the only outfit in the United States that teaches wing walking now.

Teeth or midair transfers don't figure into the curriculum at Mason Wing Walking, with the website also politely assuring readers that no student has ever fallen from the plane. But Cynthia did not want to be the first, so she phoned Marilyn Mason, the school's co-owner and lead instructor, to find out more about the physical strength and agility needed. Cynthia soon signed up. For the next six months, "I started working out in earnest," Cynthia recalls. Even when she tweaked her rotator cuff, she didn't despair. "I spent April to August getting my shoulder ready."

The wing walking decision starts making more sense when Cynthia tells me more about herself: At twenty-one, she'd

wanted to learn to skydive, but it was 1969 and a sport domi-
nated by men, mostly ex-military. "Nobody wanted to teach
me," Cynthia recalls. "Except one guy. And I ended up
marrying him!" She jumped until she was pregnant with her
first child. She continued to be active—she and her husband
hiked, camped, bicycled. He encouraged her independence,
"which was good because I wouldn't have married him otherwise." They raised daughters and spent as much time as possible
outside. Cynthia had only finished high school ("My grades
were so bad"), so at twenty-six she began college for an associate degree in electronics, then studied math. She ultimately
graduated, at age forty-four. She'd taught computer classes
throughout; then, at forty-seven years old, she took a job
with an aerospace company. "It was unusual to hire an engi-
neer that late in one's life. I was lucky. I was the only woman
for a long time. I didn't take any crap off of the guys. But
mostly they were really nice to me. Hell, they needed me."

When her husband died, in 2014, Cynthia put her independence to the true test. She was a widow now, and battling
cancer. "I was going to the gym, lifting weights, but I knew
by the time I was sixty-eight I was going to lose strength every
year." The things she loved would be falling away; she needed
to take full advantage. "I had to get out there and get this stuff
done!" she tells me.

She was still mountain biking, for example, but after the
cancer treatments, her skills deteriorated. "When I went out
to ride again, I fell, and I thought, Uh-oh, I'm not doing so
good here. Then I fell again and cracked some ribs. I said,
Okay, God, I hear you." She switched to road biking at sixty-
eight. "You just keep changing, altering the activities you
want to do so you can keep doing them."

One by one though, activities had to fall away. Today she sounds philosophical about it. She stopped snowboarding in her late sixties ("I didn't have the stamina; after two hours I was exhausted"), but she muses that she had already done it for so many years, she had no regrets. The same with scuba, which she let go of after the energy-sapping cancer treatments. "Twenty-nine years was good!" she tells me.

When it came time for her wing walking class, Cynthia arrived a day early. She camped at a nearby KOA campground, then went to observe the class. She wanted to quietly assess whether she was mentally and physically capable. To her, attending and then quitting halfway through because her nerves or her shoulder couldn't hack it would be the worst. But she watched the class from the side of the hangar and knew she was ready. The next day, she began her training. The bulk of the seminar, Cynthia tells me, is spent going over each handhold and foot move between the snug safety of the cockpit and the click of the harness that belts you to the post on the wing. "We practiced like seventy-five times each," Cynthia says. What they couldn't practice for was the fact that these moves would be executed at an altitude of thirty-five hundred feet, while the plane was flying. But Mason Wing Walking's philosophy is that if you repeat the moves while land-bound, the sequence becomes second nature in the air.

Marilyn Mason told Cynthia early on that most of the people who don't ultimately complete their wing walk are those who hesitate while in the cockpit. So when the plane was high above the ocean, the cliffs a thin pencil line and the green fields just squares on a chess set, and Mike Mason, Marilyn's husband and the pilot, indicated it was time, Cynthia shot right up. She wove her way around the cables, plodding through each move she'd learned. She says that the concentration required meant that she wasn't really registering the whole experience yet: that it was thousands of feet to the ground, that there was nothing around her, that she was *climbing on a wing, for God's sake*. Still, somewhere in her brain, alongside the neurons firing muscles and tendons, were neurons that were applauding. "When I first grabbed the handhold and stood up and put my foot on the seat . . . after that I just knew, of course I could do this. You can't imagine the confidence you're building once you're up there."

. . .

This is why one stormy day I find myself at Mason Wing Walking Academy, milling around a large red biplane and fiddling with a climbing harness. In search of this elusive confidence, I am right now learning to buckle and unbuckle the belt from various angles (in front of me as well as behind my back). The large hangar is cold, and we can hear the rain thrumming on the roof. The forecast promises that the skies will clear at least intermittently at a certain time, so Marilyn, our instructor, is watching the clock as well as our technique. There are two other students with me today: Lindley, age fifty-four, Caucasian, is a boxy military veteran who owns a cleaning company and tells us that he absolutely hates heights and has no idea why he is doing this to himself. Meir, on the other hand, is clearly not nervous at all. The youngest of us by far, at thirty-five, African American, she bought these lessons as a birthday present to herself. Both Lindley and Meir exchange skydiving stories. Lindley has also BASE jumped, which makes Meir's eyes light up; soon they are trading BASE jumping class information, too. When I ask Meir why she

wants to wing walk today, she says simply, "I'm a daredevil."
Lindley nods and agrees that he is, too.

Listening to my two cohorts, I wonder where I land on
that "daredevil" spectrum these days. When I was young I
welcomed inane exploits, like jumping into quarries and
climbing bridges. I paraglided when it was a new sport, the
equipment in its nascent stages. (A few years after I stopped
paragliding, a friend of mine decided to learn. I gifted him
my gear, including the wing itself, which I deemed the paraglider equivalent of a minivan. His instructor forbade its use,
proclaiming its rudimentary design "a death trap.") I picked
jobs like white water raft guide and eventually big-city firefighter. For all intents and purposes, I sure looked like a
daredevil.

But the truth is, that person barreled through life with a
clenched jaw. She wasn't a show-off, but she had a lot to prove.
She didn't seem to be enjoying herself a lot of the time. She
wasn't comfortable in her skin. And she was, like many young
people, sure she knew all about life, when actually she understood very little.

Luckily, I've slowly learned, and I like the person I have
become. However, I am dismayed by what seems to be a new
and unfamiliar disinterest in daredevilry. I can't tell if it's the
sedating effect of the pandemic, or just the normal evolution
of aging, or perhaps something particular to my own growth
as a person. All I know is that I'm no longer as piqued by
adrenaline. Roller coaster ride? No, thank you. Big white
water? I'll pass. Night in, with my wife next to me and cats
on my lap? Definitely.

The adventures I do engage in—stand-up paddling, say,
or even getting on my Onewheel—offer a sense of calm, not

excitement. Many people don't believe me, but even flying experimental aircraft isn't an adrenaline sport for me; upon return from a flight I am much more liable to wax poetic about the color of the sky than exclaim about a dicey crosswind. Such an obvious slide in my status from daredevil to something else yet unnamed has been leaving me confused, even ashamed—am I getting boring as I age? Am I giving in to a soporific later life? Whatever is going on, the upshot is that today I am not bright-eyed like Meir, nor am I hopped up on fear and adrenaline like Lindley. I am still murky on the point of getting out of a perfectly good cockpit and securing oneself to the top of a wing, a position that looks close to being tied to a funeral pyre. But Cynthia's experience has made me curious; I'd like to decipher what wing walking as a novel activity might offer the aging body and neural system.

It turns out that wing walking class is more about clambering, crouching, slithering, and panting than any sort of walking. But the gist, which Marilyn Mason explains to the three of us, is to memorize the sequence that guides us from cockpit to wing to post, not just with our brain but with our body. As Cynthia had explained to me and Marilyn now reiterates, we would be practicing over and over, until each movement was locked into muscle memory. The idea, I gather, is that the part of the brain that would normally scream *What the hell are you doing here?* would instead be linking to tendons and muscles in a friendly, banal conversation: "Oh, that foot there, yes, please, then this hand here." It's worth mentioning that there is also a safety cable that attaches us from our harness to the plane. But there is no instruction on what to do if we do find ourselves dangling from a strut in midair, and no one brings it up.

We practice for the next few hours. Marilyn, fifty years old, is a wing walker herself; she performs for the annual air show in town and, she tells me, gets on a wing "a few times a year, just for the fun of it." She is also a very competent instructor, knowing when to correct—Left foot first! Wrap the elbow around the cable like a chicken wing!—and when to leave us to tangle ourselves in the cables, extricate, and start over. The one thing we can't practice for, of course, is the altitude. How will it feel to be slinking onto a wing while up so high? Part of me wonders why we can't just attach ourselves to the post before takeoff and dispense with the walking part altogether; actually, Marilyn tells us, this is how the only wing walking school in England does it. But, she adds, many of those students sign up for a Mason Wing Walking experience afterward, as if just being along for a ride does not provide true fulfillment. Turns out personal agency—manifested in not just the perambulation part, but also, say, in the months of training that Cynthia embarked on—is one of the critical but unsung moves in the whole wing walking sequence.

As the afternoon approaches, the three of us begin to exhibit a modicum of wing walking skill. We chicken-wing with grace, we buckle up with speed. When the cloud ceiling begins to lift, we agree to cut short our practice in the hope of catching the weather window. Meir offers to go first. She dons her cap and goggles, climbs into the cockpit the way we have been taught, and waves. The red biplane coughs to life. Within moments, Meir has disappeared into the gray gloom.

I am not quite sure what to expect. Meir has done so many adventurous things—how will this compare? Will she even get out of her seat and onto the wing? I suspect, yes. And sure enough, as the biplane returns I can already see Meir shaking her head and grinning. New wing walkers apparently lose much of their ability to speak in full sentences, but we get the gist of it: AMAZING. Just amazing.

As the biplane is refueled, Lindley tightens the small circles he has been pacing. I am not fooled; a key component of his adventures is to steadily corkscrew into higher and higher emotion, so that the payoff is all the more sweet. Right now, though, he honestly seems to be regretting every decision that led him here to this moment, about to wing walk. "I hate heights," he keeps saying, adding, "Sharks, too . . . Sharks and heights, I just hate them."

"I assume you surf, then," I say, half laughing, but he shakes his head vehemently.

"No way!" he cries. "Absolutely not!" He climbs into the cockpit.

The biplane disappears into the clouds. I feel my own anticipation build. I go through the wing walking steps in my head one more time. Left foot up! Hands high! Chicken wing!

When Lindley returns, the answer to whether he has completed his walk comes only after he tumbles from the cockpit and falls on the grass. Covering his face, he exclaims, "Can't even explain it! Better than BASE jumping!"

Mike, who has over thirteen thousand hours of flying, scans the sky. Should we wait a few hours? The ceiling has lowered, but within a few minutes it seems to open up again, and he is hopeful there's a hole in the cloud layer. Off we go. We skirt dark shrouds. For a second it seems as if we will have to turn back, but Mike finds his hole and suddenly the ground has disappeared; we are above a bouncy house of white. There is an eerie feeling of floating, and I want to turn and remind Mike that I am like any normal person and scared of heights, and should I really be doing this? I don't, of course, and even if I did, Mike can't hear me. We are corresponding by wing waggles and hand gestures; as a last resort, he may lean forward and tap me on the shoulder. I begin a sequence of combat breaths, inhale to the count of four, hold, exhale to the count of six. Repeat. (As James Nestor tells us in his excellent book *Breath,* inhaling slowly and deeply, then extending an equally slow exhale, stimulates nerves located in the bottom quadrant of the lung that are responsible for relaxation.)

The wing waggles. Really? It's time? I remember that Cynthia popped right up, so I do the same.

Immediately, I am hit by the wind. Hold it, how did a seventy-one-year-old not notice this ungodly blast? Didn't Cynthia *specifically* say that the wind was no big deal? I shuffle through the interview in microseconds, feeling betrayed. Yes. She definitely told me the wind was negligible. Clearly, wing walking has parallels to childbirth, where the difficult parts are forgotten and only the joy remains. I double down on concentration, looking for the first foot placement. I catch sight of the yawning chasm below. Surprisingly, my stomach doesn't lurch, nor do my knees go weak. Marilyn was right (of course)—with my neural pathways already so clogged with messages to my legs and hands, now moving like molasses against the wind, there is no room in the system to transmit abject terror. Bend knee here, now grab the cable high. No, you've gone forward too quickly, back out and do it again. Twist the body, chicken-wing the arms. There is white and blue in my periphery, and a vague sense that Mike has put the plane in a gentle climb, while I grab for the final post. This isn't fear, exactly, but I am aware that one leg is skewed far to the left, as if reaching for the safety of the cockpit. The other foot, though, makes it into the foot pad, then there is the fumble for the harness. Click, click. Multiple superhuman pulls to tighten the straps (we have been warned that any looseness around the waist won't feel good while upside down.)

I shoot a thumb out, indicating I am strapped in and ready to go.

The plane rockets skyward. As it climbs, my mind shuffles around in a state of bewilderment. It ransacks neurons and old memories for a pattern to latch on to. Too late. The horizon curdles, falls away. Spinning earth, buffeting air, iceberg clouds flashing by. The sensation of falling. Shreds of green between the white. Plosives of thought—*danger, danger,* the brain insists, even as it registers the tight strap, the pilot with his thirteen thousand hours of competence. The clouds shatter and regroup. There is a cartwheeling of feet overhead. Blues and greens catapult away. At one point the coastline becomes clear. I register that we've executed a loop, then another. The view is beautiful and dreamlike—undulating cloud layers on all sides, the peaks of the Olympic Mountains jutting through. Colors of slate and blue. My brain stabilizes enough to take this in, but now it's the hammerhead move: the aircraft ascends steadily, only to lose interest at the top. There is a moment of weightlessness, then the plane falls to one side. We are plummeting to earth again. I am no longer afraid. I am something else entirely. Oddly, I begin to laugh.

What I'm experiencing, I later realize, is textbook *awe.* The awe state is an emotion, the psychologist and author Dacher Keltner explains, "in the upper reaches of pleasure and on the boundary of fear." Dread (yes), expansiveness, veneration, a sense of mystery—these are also all awe traits, "elicited when in the presence of vast things not immediately understood," as a recent study states on the matter. This is a clunky explanation, but that is apt—awe is often beyond the reach of suitable words, even for academics and scientists. Suffice it to say that awe, once only associated with religious epiphanies, is shown to be triggered by any novel experience. Like, say, wing walking.

Research on awe has exploded recently, because awe is not only, well, awesome, it is also good for you. In her book *The Extended Mind*, Annie Murphy Paul says that when we are awestruck, "we become more curious and openminded. And we become more willing to update . . . the templates we use to understand ourselves and the world." Paul points out that as a culture we are badly in need of awe. Our technologies have brought most uncertainty to heel, and even our phone is an anti-awe device, its small screen size training us to think small, while it "enlarges and aggrandizes our sense of self." Conversely, the process of awe "makes us feel tiny, even as it opens wide our sense of the possible."

I recognize how perfectly wing walking primes us for awe: there is the majestic view at thirty-five hundred feet that feels almost religious; there is the total disequilibrium of doing something so antithetical to every survival instinct; there is the exhilaration of twirling and ricocheting and falling in a vast sky. I had come to Mason Wing Walking to evaluate the confidence I might feel from the courage it took to wing walk, but instead realize that it is awe that makes the adventure so impactful.

There may be many ways to induce awe—music, poetry, the leap of a ballet dancer—but nature's vastness—what Paul calls "the unfathomable scale of the ocean, of the mountains, of the night sky"—is a surefire awe trigger. "Our everyday experience does not prepare us to assimilate the gaping hugeness of the Grand Canyon or the crashing grandeur of Niagara Falls . . . we have no response at the ready; our usual frames of reference don't fit . . . [which is why] the experience of awe has been called a 'reset button' for the human brain."

Everyday experience does not prepare for the act of wing walking, either. No wonder my mind feels blown. And something else strikes me: Could this be what has really been motivating my outdoor quests these past few years? Instead of adrenaline, have I unwittingly been seeking awe? This would mean that I was, as suspected, not really a daredevil. But I also wasn't boring, or giving up as I aged. I was instead inadvertently opening my mind and changing my perspective. I was seeking more, not less, from life in this later stage.

Turns out, you don't have to wing walk to experience awe. You can dispense with the wing entirely and simply walk, according to researchers from the Memory Care and Aging Institute at the University of California, San Francisco, who decided to send volunteers between the ages of sixty and ninety on what they called awe walks. Virginia Sturm, neurology professor at UCSF, led the study, asking these volunteers to amble outside for fifteen minutes a week while "looking at everything with fresh, childlike eyes." The idea was to attempt to "cultivate awe" by asking walkers to look closely at the natural beauty along the way. It struck me as I read this that Dot had taken me on this kind of walk, navigating as she did without a map, her waypoints only the wonder of a tree, her love of someone else's backyard, her curiosity about the color of a leaf. Birding, too, accessed awe, as we perked our ears to possibility and widened our eyes, ready for the next surprise. Certainly, I couldn't forget how I stood gobsmacked by the sight of the pearlescent green heron skimming across the pond—that feeling was awe, plain and simple.

The UCSF awe walkers soon began to notice a sustained difference in their moods. They reported upticks in well-being after each walk, but even more than that, they found that any underlying depression and anxiety noticeably retreated; emotions like gratitude and compassion rose instead, even after the awe walk study was over (inflammation—a symptom of ill health—also fell significantly). Meanwhile a control group, who strolled without the advice to pay close attention to their surroundings, spent much of their walk time in a way recognizable to most of us—ruminating on to-do lists and plans. These walkers reported no change in baseline depression, anxiety, gratitude, or compassion. Sturm says, "What we show here is that a very simple intervention—essentially a reminder to occasionally shift our energy and attention outward instead of inward—can lead to significant improvements in emotional well-being."

Still, awe walks seem qualitatively different from a wing walk. No awe walkers wind themselves up into a fear frenzy, nor do their brains have to grapple with apparent signs of imminent death during a loop and a hammerhead. The walker-on-paths has to be reminded to see things anew, while the wing walker is catapulted into that mindset. Yet the amazement is real for both.

What exactly is going on? The scientists noticed that as the awe walks progressed over the eight-week time period, the selfies that each volunteer had been asked to provide for each walk began to change. They centered their own faces less and less and allowed the backdrops to take over, what the researchers began to call a "small self" perspective. (The selfies also showed what was described in science-speak as "increasing smile intensity.") Sturm says that this shift signals "a healthy sense of proportion between your own self and the bigger picture of the world around you." In other words, less preoccupation with our own lives makes space for a wider understanding of what's outside of us, and our interconnectedness, producing generosity and generally prosocial behavior (in one seemingly banal but effective study, researchers saw that people who gazed up at towering old-growth trees were afterward very likely to help pick up pens that a stranger dropped on the ground).

The acrobatics are over. For a few minutes we fly straight and level, and I savor this, too. Then the wing waggles; I begin the slow and careful process of retreating to the cockpit. Unbuckle, reach out foot, cling to guide wire. Look down if you want! (No, don't.) Reverse chicken-wing. Reverse twist. Step back, flail the foot in the air, find the spot. Breathe, slide into the seat. Mike turns for home.

When the biplane lands and comes to a stop next to the expectant faces of my newfound compatriots, I too don't have words, so I recycle what everyone else has said. "Wow! Whoa! Amazing!" Meanwhile, my body is there on the tarmac, but my spirit is still barrel-rolling in the sky.

. . .

After this experience, I look deeper. I find studies by Paula Williams, a psychologist at the University of Utah, that show another powerful attribute of awe: emotional resilience. People with the ability to feel awe, she says, are also those who end up telling helpful stories about themselves. Never was that more clear than while I was hiking around the Grand Canyon years ago. At the time the incident puzzled me, but now it made absolute sense.

My hiking partner and I were fit and in our thirties; the walk to the floor of the canyon wasn't super challenging. But it was tiring in its own way: it was a steady downhill, but nine miles of downhill, and the terrain was pocked with rocks and loose soil, so that each step required a quick assessment—was this the right spot? Would I slip? Along the path were weather-beaten signposts, of mile numbers, of forking trails, and of reminders that overnight camping was prohibited—you had to make it all the way down to the canyon floor or go back up. I remember being so happy to reach the bottom, and thinking uneasily about the hike up and out.

We arrived at the place where we were staying, a rustic camp of old cabins and areas to place tents. There we met an older woman who I guessed to be in her late seventies at the time, but now I think it was more likely that she was in her early sixties. I remember vividly how thrilled she was to be there. She rhapsodized about the towering cliff faces, the wildlife, this once-in-a-lifetime opportunity. *"The Grand Canyon!"* she kept saying, as if she couldn't believe she was standing on its golden soil, peering at its majestic shoulders. I was tickled by her lit-up face, her spilling-over enthusiasm. But I was also puzzled. She used a cane, limped, and was quickly out of breath when she walked. How had she arrived? There were no roads, no cars. Had she come in by mule? "Oh, no," she said. "I walked the trail." She relayed this to me with pride, and I could see why. The walk had been long and my legs were tired. And to do it with a cane? I was agog.

She seemed to read my mind. No, she had never done anything like this before, she said. But it had been fantastic. "But of course I was so slow." She sweeps one arm at herself, as if to say, Look at me, after all. "So we didn't make it down and we had to sleep on the path." She and her companion (I can't remember if it was her husband or a friend) had no sleeping bags. There was only one of those metallic silver sheets, billed as an emergency blanket, and the ponchos they'd packed for the rain. Their water was gone, and so were their trail peanuts. "It was so cold," she said. A ranger came by at sundown and saw them sitting down. He said it was against park rules to stop, but what could he do? This woman with the cane wasn't going to get teleported the remaining few miles. He gave them some more water and left.

So she spent a long and freezing night on the trail. I imagined the many miserable hours of no sleep and half sleep, barely protected from the cold desert environment, then the many hours the next day of continuing descent. Yet here she was, beatific.

"Luckily you can take mules back up," I said to her. She looked at me as if I were crazy. The ranger had offered her that, too, she said, but no, she wanted to walk it. That was the real way to experience the Grand Canyon, she said. The park service, however, was stern, pretty much telling her that they would be billing her the hundreds of thousands of dollars any rescue would cost, and she left the canyon by mule. Her story was clearly a cautionary tale about responsibility in the outdoors, about risk assessment, about understanding limits. But what really stayed with me was this woman's enthusiasm. She hadn't been cowed by her misadventure. She'd been invigorated. What I felt in her presence was the irrepressible happiness of someone who had experienced the mind-boggling beauty and challenge of a wilderness adventure. She was absolutely radiant with it.

This ability to extricate a positive narrative from a scrum of possible, excruciatingly negative versions is an attitude that is vital as we face the rigors of life and eventually of older age. This stranger so many years ago never complained about her situation. Instead, subsumed by awe, she was extolling it.

. . .

Dr. Louise Aronson points out in her book *Elderhood* that as a culture we mostly refuse to embrace this last stage of life. Each of us will one day arrive here (that dismissive auto mechanic, or the young usher at the concert who doesn't bother looking your way—remember that they too will be old soon enough). Yet instead of accepting older age, Dr. Aronson points out, we are trying to cure it. Plastic surgery is just one symptom of that. So are the many longevity studies uninterested in improving aging, only in skirting it altogether.

What if more of us embraced awe? Wouldn't the ensuing years, with their increasing wisdom, become something rejuvenating and exciting?

Behold, says the Christian Bible, over and over. *Behold.* What is "behold" but a directive to look closely and be amazed? Religion has long taught its faithful to be open to awe, and I wonder where Cynthia's own religious background intersects with her experiences outdoors. She has invoked God multiple times in our conversations, and when I ask, she affirms that she grew up Catholic. In these later years, she's given up going to church, but she keeps her relationship with God, she tells me.

During the hammerhead maneuver, just before the plane dropped sideways, Cynthia remembers yelling out, "I'm alive!" She wasn't experiencing adrenaline, she says, so she supposes it was awe that triggered the outburst. "I was so happy," she tells me. Honestly, I get the sense that Cynthia is often overcome, and it doesn't have to coincide with acrobatics in the sky. "When I take my dog for a walk and it's night and all the stars come out, I just take a deep breath and feel so much joy. I think, Thank you, God, for giving me such a wonderful life." When she sees people in her senior residence using walkers, and contemplates her own relatively healthy state, she tells God she is grateful. Even during her toughest moments, when her husband passed away and she battled cancer, she retained not just her faith, but her appreciation. Dying didn't scare her, she says, or make her angry, because she'd had such a full, rewarding life. The process was yet another adventure, not exactly found on Google under "Something fun to do here," but an experience she wanted to face with grace. She tells me that when her survival was in doubt during her cancer battle, she prayed, "Hey, God, don't let me be a wimp. I want to go out with courage." It strikes me that this ability to feel gratitude and optimism in the face of difficulty is exactly what Williams's studies on awe have shown. Perhaps Cynthia was born with this trait. However, adventure, and the awe it inspires, could only have deepened it.

Cynthia asks me if I have advice on what to investigate next, but then answers her own question before I can offer any ideas. "You know what I want to do? Dragon boating. I should look that up . . ." Her voice trails off as if she is already stepping away from the phone conversation and sling-shotting to the day when she will drop herself into the large dragon-shaped canoe and nod to her fellow boating enthusiasts, who have also embraced this obscure racing sport. She will pull on her paddle in time with her teammates, feel the wind in her hair, the spray of the ocean, her God nearby. I hear her add, as if speaking to herself, "There's only so many years of life left, so, by gum, let's do it."

BRAIN

7

Learn Something New

It's great to suck at something.

—Karen Rinaldi, fifty-five, surfer, who learned
the sport later in life (and proudly sucks at it)

One fine winter day, I sit on my surfboard in thick fog. I can't see the beach, but I know that it's behind me, because the wave faces are rolling in and breaking, sometimes on my head. I've caught one or two, but all inelegantly. Nearby is my fellow writer and friend, Bonnie Tsui, more than a decade younger than me, a much better surfer, her yellow helmet a blurry beacon. Every now and then a dark figure comes into focus—another intrepid human on a board—and then disappears back into the gloom. I feel spectral, the outer edges of me dissolving into water and air, and I'm intermittently sure that Bonnie and I are the only two people in the world, if this is indeed the world, which it doesn't feel like. It is instead some liminal space where reality meets unreality, and then waits. Meanwhile, incoming waves lurch out of the fog in slow, lethargic succession. Maneuvering to meet each one, I watch my hands cup the ocean; the sudden bracing cold on my skin and the thin lace of water I flick into the air reminds me that I do indeed exist.

At the end of the session we paddle toward what we know is the beach, but can't see. Even when we walk up onto the sand we don't know where we are. Usually there is a cityscape behind the dunes, rectangles and spires in plain view. Now every feature is erased. We know only that we are not where we had begun; this is a surf spot with a reputation for pulling surfers as much as a half mile along the shore on what seems like a whim (tidal flow and swell direction are a factor, but so is the shifting topography of the ocean floor). We want to return to our cars, parked along the frontage road. Should we head to the left or to the right? We have no idea.

We stand there for a little while debating (me: I think left because the tide is coming in. Bonnie: I think right. I have a feeling.) We finally see a shadow emerge from the gloom and trudge by us. Another surfer, heading right. Does he know what he is doing? When a second ghost materializes, takes shape, and passes us heading right again, we shrug and follow. Right is correct, it turns out.

We weren't in any danger that day. We would have found our cars eventually. But for a little while the world was murky and indistinct. With that came a feeling of surrender—no matter how much I strained my eyes, I couldn't see through the fog. There was also a faint anxiety, but this was pushed aside by the alertness that comes with a new predicament. I was at once floating in the brume and firmly rooted in the moment. Scientists call this sensation "psychological disequilibrium." Our senses are knocked about, as well as our feelings—there's a little fear, a lot of exhilaration. That day my own synapses were valiantly trying to make sense of the situation, offering a thrum of words that assured me that this murky veil would lift . . . or would it? Only a few hours before, my brain had been a hurtling train on its usual commuter schedule, but suddenly a lever had been pulled, the synaptic route disrupted. The mechanism that switched tracks slowly trundled into place, and now the whole landscape was different. Meanwhile, the neurological conductor ran to the forward car to frantically rifle through itineraries. Where was the next station now?

Psychological disequilibrium, the research says, is what allows for growth and change both neurologically and emotionally. And the outdoors is full of the uncertainties needed for a brain to grow. The weather changes, the hill is steeper than we thought. We forget the matches, the chocolate (heaven forbid). Now we, and our brains, have to make do. No wonder some parents throw their disconsolate teens into wilderness programs, sure that rain, steep hikes, menacing fauna, and expansive views can do in one month what years of therapy or parental discipline cannot. Outdoor adventure works for young people; why can't it work for older people, too?

. . .

San Manuel Airport—also known as E77, or Echo Seven Seven in pilot speak—has been flight instructor Britta Penca's home base for a few years now. Right now, I'm above this pretty little Arizona airport, looking at the ground with something like the longing of a puppy for her mother. The experimental aircraft I'm in is bobbling from side to side, the stick in my hand hard to control. From my vantage point seven hundred feet above the runway, I have a clear view of the windsock jerking and spinning, just as the automated weather station intones wind speed into our headsets with the gravity of some robotic god. *Ah, my mortal minions, welcome to my shitstorm. Behold, a crosswind gusting to twenty knots.*

I can feel my brain starting to fracture with textbook psychological disequilibrium.

Britta's reaction to all this is unclear—she's seated behind me—but there's no indication that she's aware that this particular flying machine, called a gyrocopter, is not meant to land in a crosswind of over twenty-five knots, a mere five knots away from present conditions. Instead, her voice is calm. She tells me she's taking the controls. "You have the controls," I answer, obeying the protocol that aviation students repeat what the instructor says. For goodness' sake, please, have them, stammers my disequilibrium-ing mind.

Britta dips the aircraft into a steep turn. There is no glass canopy locking us in, and for a moment it feels as if I might be dislodged from my seat and then drop like a stone to the earth below. She abruptly levels out, but the boxing match doesn't stop: hot air popping off from the desert floor jabs and hooks; the aircraft bucks and weaves in response. Meanwhile, the runway widens in the windshield; instinctively I lean back. Being in the front seat without the controls does not come easily to a seasoned pilot, so I'm grinding my teeth, forcing myself not to grab anything with my hands or push anything with my feet. Then we're skimming the ground, the large runway numbers flashing underneath us. It looks like a perfect touchdown. But at the last second, we are pushed sideways. In my sightline, the runway twists. A snarl of engine rpms: Britta has hit the throttle. We lift quickly into the air. We've aborted the landing.

"Well, this might take ten times, but bear with me," Britta tells me over the headset. The normal human being in me recoils just a little. But the pilot in me is pretty thrilled. "No problem," I say, and it's true. Britta is a very, very good aviator and the machine we are in is as nimble as a cutting horse. She begins the turn for another try.

. . .

A few months ago, I asked myself what seemed at the time a simple question: Could I, at fifty-seven years old, learn something new? It had been a long time (wing walking was still in my future at this point) since I had set my mind to a set of really immersive new skills. Years, really, if you didn't count learning how to stand six feet from people at all costs during the pandemic that had hit nine months before and still had the world firmly in its unforgiving grip.

The ensuing lockdown meant that many adults were getting forcibly reacquainted with the Roman Empire, sentencing diagramming, and algebra, as those who were not frontline workers stayed at home and tried to tutor their children. Others tackled a new, in-depth understanding of Zoom for their jobs, now conducted from a cramped room in their house. There was sourdough baking. There were TikTok dances. But none of that interested me. I had been mulling a certain skill for a while. It wasn't completely foreign, yet would still require some large neural resets and challenges—some good old psychological disequilibrium.

I wanted to fly a gyrocopter.

The gyrocopter is a strange machine, with the silhouette of a wasp and a name that sounds like a disease one might catch in the tropics. Yes, I was already an experienced pilot. I had learned to fly fixed-wing aircraft, specifically Cessnas, when I was twenty; I turned to paragliding in my thirties. For the past fifteen years, I have flown a motorized hang glider, also known as a "trike" because of the three landing wheels tacked onto what otherwise looks like a riding lawn mower that dangles from a hang glider wing. Still, a gyro was different from these other aircraft. It had characteristics of both a helicopter and a plane, with a large rotor on the top and a propeller behind (thus some called it a gyrocopter, others a gyroplane), yet it was neither. It was the *Equus mulus* of aircraft, in that liminal space between a donkey and a horse, not wholly one, not wholly the other. This was fitting because I was fifty-seven years old, not young but not old, either. It was the perfect leap to take.

. . .

Does flying a machine count as outdoor adventure? It turns out that piloting a bare-bones, open-cockpit aircraft is about as close to being a bird as you will get (except if you ditch the engine altogether and use just a wing and your own feet to launch, which I did as a paraglider pilot). It's decidedly not optimal to fly by fossil fuel, though gyros use car gas and are relatively efficient (unlike, say, commercial flights that run on aviation fuel), and electric gyros are on the horizon, we are told. Moral quandaries abound, for sure. Overall, though, it must be noted that the experimental gyrocopter aircraft has little in the way of actual "craft" and much more in the way of "air"; you perch on a seat with only a low and flimsy carbon fiber foot bed that rises no more than knee height, and a nose cone for aerodynamics that allows for a small windshield and some rudimentary instruments nestled into a forward panel. Other than that, you are intimately a part of any weather system you encounter, so that you obsessively pore over local conditions on various apps and government sites before you finally step outside the hangar. You swivel your head to clock the soaring birds, examine the clouds, check the tree sway, study the windsock for wind direction, decode the temperature at altitude, and make your decision. Once in the air, the earth unfolds below you like the finest, most expansive park in the world, and it's yours to hike, only this time from the height and perspective of a hawk, making the endeavor—in my opinion—both outdoorsy and adventurous in the most essential senses of the words, from the get-go.

But hold on. Was it smart to learn to fly a gyrocopter at my age? Like many women, I had gone through my early fifties with a body that seemed to betray me daily. Perimenopause had caught me by surprise. What I had been expecting at this time of life was to be "losing my menstrual period," but no one had mentioned that I would be crying suddenly and for little reason, that my brain would insist that sleep was stupid and that pacing the kitchen and eating stale tortillas was better, and that I would experience a general loss of memory, including, worst of all, an inability to identify faces, which caused me embarrassment and lots of "Hey . . . you" salutations at social engagements. When actual menopause finally happened—technically, the complete absence of one's menstrual cycle for a whole year—it was a relief. But the effects of perimenopause lingered. It had cut into my confidence. Furthermore, didn't our brains harden as we aged? Was it even neurologically possible to take on cognitive challenges? As I neared sixty, surely my brain was on par with an heirloom Christmas ornament—round, tarnished, easily broken when dropped. Something to be handled carefully, with limited uses. Could I do this?

Aging has long been proclaimed a constant diminution, not just of muscle mass, reproductive hormones, eyesight, and skin tone, but of the brain as well. As you aged, the theory went, the brain shrunk. Corners folded in. Synapses blinked out like cheap lights. And it happened early. Thinkers and scientists from Freud to Piaget claimed that brain growth ended in our early twenties, and then we were fixed there. All that could be done was to cling as desperately as possible to what we had; then, as we aged, our handhold steadily slipped, like a climber on a slowly crumbling wall, until it broke away completely, tumbling us into the void of dementia and ill health.

Since I'm on a roll, here's another belabored metaphor: Old dogs, it is said, can't learn new tricks. And they are rapidly losing the old tricks, too.

Except this is complete and utter hogwash.

As more recent research shows, the brain continually grows, changes, and adapts as we age. We do keep learning throughout our life span. Not only do our brains build new synaptic connections, but they can create entirely new brain cells, at any age. At some point there will be a natural decline, and the brain may not be able to rely on the neural pathways it once did. But it doesn't give up; instead, our trusty control center adapts by visiting new locales for information, like some steadily expanding highway system. It's worth noting here that it was a woman who proved that the icons of science had gotten it so wrong when they proclaimed that brains calcify early and then retreat. Neuroscientist Marian Diamond was in her forties when her research showed that a human brain can grow and change even as we age; she was met with incredulity and cries of incompetence from many of her fellow (male) scientists, which receded only in the face of mounting evidence. Since Diamond's groundbreaking work, it's become clear that neural growth not only means that we keep our smarts, but the new pathways we lay down may lead to different and more innovative thinking than a younger brain produces. In other words, despite "some losses with age, such as neural regions less active in older adults than in young, . . . older adults could recruit regions of the brain to support cognitive functions in ways unlike young adults." All this brain "plasticity," as it has come to be called, flies in the face of previous scientific beliefs and, even slower to fall, our cultural ones. But believe it. Believe it as if your life depends on it. Because it does.

An enriched older brain, studies show, leads overwhelmingly to longer life, better health, and sharper cognition. So how do we prod our neurons to keep firing with enthusiasm? Research points to self-care like sleep, exercise, companionship, and reduced stress, of course. But also: "Novelty, focused attention and challenge." The more we push our neural pathways to confront new questions and conundrums, the more we keep our cognitive functions spry. In other words, when we learn something new, we nurture and energize our brain, and we live longer, healthier lives.

I decided, what the heck. I'll see for myself. I'll sign up for gyrocopter lessons.

. . .

Gyrocopters represent the very fringe of flying. There aren't many instructors, and all the ones I was told about were men, which was fine and to be expected; only a little more than 6 percent of all pilots are women, so the percentage who fly gyrocopters is no doubt well under minuscule. Then I stumbled upon a website for Britta Penca. She taught out of a tiny airport in Arizona. On the phone she was relaxed, amiable, confident. She told me that she had gone to seminary, she had been employed at crisis centers, she had worked with psychiatric patients. All this seemed perfect training for a gyrocopter instructor. Even better, it turned out she was fifty-five years old. I signed up.

Britta assured me that I could learn to fly gyros, despite being fifty-seven. "Women at any age make great pilots. There's more finesse, more presence," she said. And being an older woman? That was actually an advantage in Britta's book. We've had years of things like marriage, or children, or a big career, or just making ends meet, she explains. "Now we're turning our sights to 'What about me? What brings me joy?' Our consciousness is expanded and fine-tuned. We're more grounded, more experienced. And more confident."

It may be harder to learn when older, Britta agreed. But it isn't because my brain is less functional. It's because I have *so much experience,* so much accumulated knowledge. In other words, any difficulty I have learning the gyro will not be because I'm losing my mind with age. It will be because my head is completely full up with knowledge, leaving little space for new information. As Britta said this I imagined all the cluttered rooms in my brain, and how they would now need to be emptied for new know-how. "I guess I'll chuck those four years of college to clear some space," I nervously joked.

So now I'm here, in the front seat of Britta's gyro, getting pummeled by thermals and a mean crosswind. Britta turns for the runway like a barrel racer. My intestines shift. I command myself to slow my breathing, employing those trusty combat breaths. Britta aborts the next landing.

"Sometimes it takes a while," she says, and I can hear the shrug of her shoulders in her voice. "Luckily, we have a lot of fuel."

The next few moments consist of sink, lift, sink, lift, punctuated sometimes by a sideways shudder. These conditions are new to me—I've flown my motorized hang glider in turbulence, but I never would've allowed myself to be airborne in this weather. Gyrocopters, however, handle high winds and robust thermals very well. Still, I don't expect what I hear next in my headset from Britta: "I'm going to try to land into the crosswind, across the runway, okay?" Despite the question mark at the end of her sentence she's not asking my permission. She's warning me, because landing perpendicular to a runway is not normal business. Britta tells me later that she has actually landed this way several times in the past; winds in Arizona kick up suddenly, necessitating this kind of Plan B. Very few aircraft can perform this maneuver, though a gyro piloted by someone like Britta is evidently one of them.

My mind screams *WHAT THE HELL.* "Sure, no problem," I say instead. Before I know it, we are skimming the empty airplane parking area, with the pilot shack on one side and the hangars on the other. Ahead and perpendicular to us is the runway. Her plan, I can now see, is to stay headed into the wind (which is how the aircraft wants to land; gyrocopters need runway to both take off and return) for as long as possible and then . . . touch down using the width of the runway only? Turn radically and use the length of the runway? I'm not sure. Things are losing their meaning right now. Just as we pass low over the taxiway, I hear her say *Darn.*

Darn?

Darn?

The throttle roars, the gyro quickly gains altitude, once again we have aborted. "Wind shifted again," Britta sighs. I laugh, a little wildly. The truth is that, despite my nerves, I am also having what might be called . . . fun. The air may be unpredictable, but the gyro is nimble and my instructor is unflappable. I settle in to try to really enjoy whatever happens next.

Britta lines up for a normal runway landing now. She aims for midfield. It's our sixth—or is it the seventh?—attempt. She keeps the gyro a few feet above the asphalt for a long time, then there is a slight stickiness, a hesitation in the speed that I finally recognize as the most gentle of touchdowns. Britta has set us onto the ground as if there were no crosswind at all.

"Amazing," I whisper into the headset.

She answers with a small laugh, "I was just waiting for one I liked."

Later, she explains that she wanted me to understand that just because you are on final approach, it doesn't mean you should actually land. The mental (and emotional!) ability to perform what we call in pilot lingo a *go-around* is vital for good piloting. Judging wind conditions is a skill. Aborting the landing is a skill. Fighting the urge to land at all costs—the term of art for this is get-on-the-ground-itis—is a skill. Unbeknownst to me, but now very clear, Britta had been demonstrating these important tenets. *Never take a bad landing* is the lesson today.

Learning is difficult for any brain, but trying to absorb novel information while also going mano a mano with anxiety, confusion, and a shifting digestive system can cause some short-circuiting. There is a line between shaking up the neural network to make space for new connectors and freaking out so much that it just shuts down. In the coming days, we simply land before the weather becomes too rowdy. But the extreme psychological disequilibrium I experience today has been enough to change my baseline perspective for good. I've seen what a gyro can do in a maelstrom with the right pilot at the helm. I will be less and less unnerved each time the winds kick up. Even if it takes seven attempts, I will make sure that my landing is always one that I like.

. . .

Britta is a gregarious Caucasian woman with a constant smile and two small, charming, blond braids poking out from under a gray cap. Her childhood was spent in Iowa on the family farm, running through fields and caring for the animals, with no exposure at all to aviation. When she was in her late twenties she was invited to a cookout at the local airport. Seeing her enthusiasm for the planes taking off and landing, a friend gifted her a few lessons in a Cessna. Immediately, flying spoke to her. But after a few lessons, Britta knew she would never be able to afford an airplane, so she stopped. Then, when she was thirty-four, Britta saw a gyrocopter, and her fascination with flying reignited. You could buy a gyrocopter for the price of a good motorcycle. It flew on inexpensive car gas. What the hell, if she could save the money, she would buy it and fly for fun. Which she did. But part of her felt selfish. Shouldn't she be flying for the good of something or someone? There was a brief period where she sank her savings into helicopter lessons, with a plan to work in medical evacuations. But the school abruptly folded, and with it went her money and dreams (she did obtain her helicopter license, and she has a fixed-wing license, too). Soon, however, friends began clamoring for her to become a gyrocopter instructor.

The office Britta shares with her husband, Mark, looks out onto the one runway at San Manuel Airport. Across the way is the pilot shack, that base of operations found in every small airport, just a one- or two-room shed, complete with a coffeepot, a bathroom, and a long center table, where once pilots spread out paper aeronautical charts and schemed and dreamed their next flight. (Nowadays, with GPS, this is no longer needed, though I often carry these paper maps along with my GPS, being an old-school pilot.) The decor is predict-able: planes, planes, planes. Photos of planes, calendars of planes, and models of planes, all tacked to walls or dangling from ceiling space. Here the inevitable print of the sexy woman next to a plane. There the bookcase scattered with flying manuals, spy novels, and a bunch of old flying maga-zines (really old—I found one that went back fifty years to 1971) falling into the worn-out Barcalounger that's next to the mangy velveteen sofa. Pilot shacks are so similar that if I accidentally walked into a wormhole, of which there are supposedly many here in Arizona, and was dropped into one on the opposite side of the country without notice, I would nevertheless quickly figure out that I was at a small airport in the United States of America.

Britta says that being an older woman has never been much of an issue for her business. Sometimes a student will walk in and assume Mark is the instructor (he isn't—he handles maintenance of the gyros). "Maybe some are hesitant, but [once in the air] I'm good at talking with people to let them know I'm with them, I got this, this isn't my first rodeo," she tells me. Her students don't tend to underestimate her, she says, but they do underestimate the aircraft. "They think the gyro is easy and won't take much training, and I don't feel that way."

Meanwhile I am an average student, and it does feel harder to learn. But I realize I am also much more assiduous, wanting not to miss anything, understanding that in the past there had somehow always been gaps in my learning. As a young person I took for granted my ability to assimilate information and then didn't notice, until years later, when I was puzzling over an icon on a flight chart, that some of it had never sunk in. Or perhaps I had postured too successfully, giving my instructors a false belief that I was a quicker student than I actually was, and they had skimmed through areas of knowledge that deserved more attention. Certainly, I felt pressure as one of the few females in a male-dominated arena. I first learned to fly in 1981, subsidized by my parents' generosity and a summer job as a newspaper photographer. At the time, I knew of no other female pilots (besides Amelia Earhart, of course) and I was sure it was up to me to disprove the invisible prejudgments and doubts that may or may not have been lurking there. Not only would this have been a big distraction and taken up needed brain space, but the actual act of pretending to learn quickly and seamlessly can only come back to bite. Thankfully, those years are long gone and I have little to prove. I don't care what my instructor thinks of me now. I only care about flying my new aircraft safely and with skill. Here is the revelation that also comes pretty quickly: Free of the insecurity and brainless swagger of youth, success looks different. It's not acing a test in record time, it's actually learning the material so it is of use later. On this go-round, I give everything more attention. No wonder learning feels harder. *Say that again about the rotor. One second, let me write down those airspeeds. Excuse me, can you repeat that?*

Pilots like to point out that flying is easy, it's the takeoffs and landings that are hard. They are mostly referring to the technical skill it takes to bargain with the forces of both gravity and lift, but they are also pointing to something more ethereal. When landing a plane, a pilot feels both relief and the unmistakable letdown of becoming once more that land-bound creature she was born as. There are whiffs of the regretful prodigal son returning, and a need to be home where you're safe and the hearth is warm. Fittingly, landings are uncertain. And they are difficult. The takeoff, on the other hand, is much more romantic. Here, you are shot into the sky, heading toward the heavens, leaving behind your earthly woes. But takeoffs have their own dark side, entailing smaller margins of error and higher stakes if something goes wrong (an engine failure on takeoff is every pilot's nightmare), and that is what we begin with today. My job right now, Britta tells me, is to keep the gyro in what is called wheel balance—the front wheel light, heading skyward, but the main wheels still on the ground, spinning down the runway. At a certain airspeed the mains will finally get airborne, too, and we can fly away. But for now, wheel balance requires constant tiny movements with my right hand on the control stick while managing the engine RPMs with my left.

It is here that I face an added glitch I am unprepared for. I had girded myself for some slower brain functions, but I hadn't factored in another aspect of learning at a later age that might get in the way: muscle memory. For fifteen years I have been flying that motorized hang glider trike; it turns out those controls are exactly opposite to the controls on a gyrocopter. Imagine you are driving forty-five miles per hour on a mountain road and suddenly some strange magnetic field or evil wizard (bear with me here) modifies your car; to turn right you now have to spin the steering wheel to the left, and vice versa. Could you do it? No.

At this moment I am stressed by the tarmac flashing underneath me; everything sensory feels scrambled. Swiftly, my instincts kick in, reverting to the familiar by wrenching the controls from my brain and putting them firmly into my muscles. And what my muscles remember are the controls of the craft I have been flying most recently: that darn trike. So, I pull on the stick when the nose is too high and, contrary to what I want, up that nose goes, even higher. Britta yells into the intercom to *lower* the nose, so I do—by pulling back even more. She yells again ("Voice is all I had, otherwise I wouldn't have raised it," she tells me later), then barks at me to cede the controls. She wrestles the stick forward, and finally, thankfully, settles all wheels to earth and slows us to a manageable speed.

I am sweating and exhausted; Britta, however, remains relaxed and good natured, unbothered by my inadvertent efforts to murder us both. What I am experiencing is "primacy in learning," Britta explains after we turn off the runway and park. I had been taught to pull back to lower the nose and push forward in order to lift it, and in times of stress and reactivity, of course, that is what I will revert to. I can change, she assures me. We can override this. I nod compliantly, but inside I am unsure.

At night, I sit on the edge of my bed practicing stick control (with a sawed-off broom handle in one hand, eyes closed, the perfect wheel balance hovering in my mind's eye) and give myself inner pep talks about my future as a gyro pilot. I'm also eager to hear more about Britta's own flying experience. Has it changed as she's gotten older? Is she, for instance, more anxious (like I seem to be)? She explains that, no, she isn't scared, just more careful, more safety conscious. "I used to do things just for the adventure. But now, I'm more tempered. Just because you can fly into a box canyon doesn't mean you should." She knows what could go wrong, how factors out of her control could take over. Her first flight instructor, Mary, was killed when the student she was teaching froze. She couldn't wrest the controls from him, and they plowed headlong into the ground.

Britta herself has experienced what is called a "catastrophic mechanical failure." That day she'd had a new student. He took the front seat; she would fly from the back seat, which is much more difficult but the norm during instruction. The takeoff was smooth, but at four hundred feet there was a great noise and a shudder and the engine quit. Britta didn't know it at the time, but the propeller hub had disintegrated. Totally disintegrated. The propeller broke off, like in some bad sci-fi movie, spun wildly in midair, caught the rotor above, and fell away. Because it was made of aluminum, the rotor didn't shatter (if it had been a composite rotor, Britta tells me, things would have been terribly different), but it did bend, making control more difficult. In addition, a fuel line sheared, and a fire began. In those first few microseconds, Britta only knew the broad strokes—bad noise, engine out—but it all added up to dire, dire straits.

Britta remembers clearly that she said, "I got it," to reassure her student. She peered over his shoulder for a landing place, and saw immediately that at this low altitude the terrain ahead was inhospitable—there was a drainage ditch with edges like teeth, there was a frontage road festooned with power lines and limned by trees. Iffy propositions, both. There was also the runway behind her, but that would mean a 180-degree turn, as well as a downwind landing. Drastic low-level maneuvers and downwind landings are both inadvisable, but so was the situation she was in. She told her student to count out the airspeed as it increased so that he would be preoccupied. Sixty, sixty-five, seventy-five . . . If she'd been in a fixed-wing, she tells me, she never would have tried to turn around, but a gyro is so much more maneuverable. She dropped the nose to load the rotors with as much energy as possible and turned for the runway. She was calm, not unnerved at all. This took seconds, milliseconds even. "All those years in crisis centers working with sexual assault survivors could have played a part," she tells me when I marvel at her cool head. Did age have something to do with it, too, I wonder? Not age, exactly, she says.

Experience. Hours and hours and hours of practice, so that she intuitively understood the gyro, how it flew, what it could do in a tricky situation.

The landing was beautiful.

"I was proud of that," she says now, laughing. Even the FAA investigators were amazed—they kept looking for damage from the touchdown, but couldn't find a single dent or stress fracture.

Will I ever learn this aircraft? I am despairing. Then, one morning, it clicks. It literally feels like that—a sudden shake and an audible sound as the gears make one final awkward attempt to mesh and then, wow, lock neatly into place. I feel a sudden rightness flowing through my arms. There is a newfound ease as my brain makes minute calculations and my body responds. Hallelujah! The old instincts used to fly my trike fall away, have been dislodged from my neural pathways, molt from my musculature. The new instincts to fly a gyro-copter are here. I skim the runway at the required height, I climb out at the right speed, I fly figure eights that look like eights and not some kindergartener's scribble. "I'm doing a happy dance back here," Britta exclaims through the headset.

I obtain my license. Turns out, I learn in the average amount of time, like an average student. My almost-sixty-year-old brain did just fine, after all. Now I am the proud part owner of a handsome yellow gyrocopter with my friend Paul, and it is parked in the hangar that once held my trike hang-glider-with-a-motor. I liked flying paragliders, and I liked flying trikes. But I am giddily in love with flying gyrocopters, a fact that amazes me. How could I become so passionate about a new endeavor at this advanced age? Aren't I supposed to be jaded? Grumpy? Sedated by a slowing endocrine system? Ah, yet another bunch of falsehoods I've been fed about growing older. Instead, I throw open the hangar doors eagerly. I carefully go through my checklist, I taxi to the runway. I key the mic and tell anyone who might be listening that the sky is about to be mine.

Embrace Disequilibrium

I don't think the feeling of regret is a negative emotion. . . .
What's negative are thoughts like I can't run fast anymore or
I'm too old to do this. . . . Use any regrets you might
have as motivation to achieve a goal.

—Mariko Yugeta, sixty-three, who is now
running faster than she did as a competitive
runner in her twenties

Diana Nyad was sixty-four when she finally swam from Cuba to the mainland United States—110 miles of currents, sharks, jellyfish, and weather—becoming the first person to do so without a shark cage. Nyad had attempted this crossing four times before, starting as early as age twenty-eight, and each time she was thwarted. Others had also tried—and been overcome by the vicious stings, storms, and currents that characterize this part of the Atlantic Ocean. This is why, when Nyad finally clambered on shaky sea legs up the Florida beach after fifty-three hours in the water—almost two and a half days—the world was awed. Not only had this woman persevered despite the specter of four previous failures. But she had the tenacity, no, the *audacity*, to think that as she got older she could hope to do better. And do better she did.

Once on the beach, she had some advice for the rest of us mere mortals, and it was worth listening to. "First, never give up. Second, you are never too old to chase your dreams . . ." She mumbled all this through lips swollen with salt, and how could we not believe her, this person who had defied reason and temperance and everything we thought we knew about aging women.

This is what I think of as I sit by another body of water, a condominium pool perched on a pretty mountainside in Pacific Palisades, California.

Because Diane Espaldon, age fifty-nine, wants to chase a dream, a dream that, to her, is also a nightmare. Diane is here to learn to swim. Not across the Atlantic. Just across this pool—that will do for now.

I watch as Diane presses goggles against her eyes, and then, as instructed, makes the surprise face to see if they fit. She wrestles the cap around her long black-gray hair. She marches to the side of the pool without hesitation and looks directly into its blue depths. Diane loves water, and still cherishes the memory of clinging to her father's back, holding her breath, and then gliding with him deep into the warm ocean depths of Guam, where he was a free diver and where she was born and grew up.

But.

Another part of Diane doesn't want to swim at all. This Diane hates the feeling of water splashing on her face. This Diane has an interior monologue that goes something like this: What the hell are you doing? You've tried to learn to swim five separate times in your life. It's never worked. You're going to drown. You're going to drown. You're going to drown. This Diane tells Ian, her instructor, that despite repeated lessons over the years, her fear has held her back from being somebody who considers herself a swimmer. "I like the feeling of being underwater. At least I did a long time ago. But there's something about being on the surface with the water splashing in my face, my eyes, and my nose."

I am at the side of the pool watching both Dianes merge into one blue bathing suit and take the first swimming lesson in years, after that string of failed attempts. I am curious if aging will make the process finally click. Possibly she and I will be disappointed and learn that aging is no magic potion, no wise arbiter of youthful fears, no sudden last-chance grantor of dreams. But that's okay. I am here because no matter what the outcome of Diane Espaldon's swimming-lesson adventure, she is learning something new, and I would like to observe that process, whether she succeeds or not. Invigorating the brain with novelty is one of the best ways to keep it sharp, as I have said. It is also a way to fend off other attributes that afflict us as the years progress—depression, for one. Low self-esteem, for another. Perhaps most important, goal setting of this sort is vital to our continued sense of purpose, which often sags as we age. This makes "success" based on outcome an inaccurate word, because Diane has already succeeded. She has dragged herself here, poolside, despite the voices, the fears, the part of her that could shrug and say, Well, I've come this far without comfort in water, why bother changing that? Instead, she is ready to try again after a lifetime of feeling as if her swimming phobia keeps winning over that part of her that actually has a deep and soulful affinity for water.

Her instructor, Ian—who is also my wonderful brother-in-law, married to my twin sister—stands nearby, putting on his own cap and goggles as he speaks with Diane, gaining an initial impression not just of her relationship to water, but who she is and how best to teach her. He has years of experience coaching professional triathletes and newbie swimmers as well as those in between—some of whom can easily freestyle many lengths of a pool but who shed all composure and technique when faced with, say, open water. Swimming, he knows, is a complex skill—done wrong it is not just physically exhausting, but it also triggers all our psychological survival responses. (If you run wrong, or even bicycle wrong, you may become tired and frustrated, or even—in the case of a careening bike— prickly with fear at points, but there is no equivalent to the deep primal need to be on dry land, the panicky hyperventilation and wild dog-paddle to shore.) Ian, himself aged fifty-two, seems to realize that while Diane has trepidation, she is also gutsy, because he doesn't launch into a soothing monologue about fears and nerves and everything-will-be-all-right. He simply asks her why she wants to learn to swim.

She tells him that first and foremost, and probably most obviously, she doesn't want to drown. Second, "I realize that there's an entire area of life I can't participate in." Also, she wants to keep up with her daughter, Lily, who is fourteen and very physically active; Diane dreams of accompanying her as she tries new things. "She goes in the ocean and I sit on the beach and say, 'Careful, honey,'" she explains with a rueful shake of her head. Top of mind for Diane, also: if Lily did find herself in trouble, struck by a sneaker wave, or dragged by a misplaced current, Diane knows she would be unable to save her.

Finally, "I'd love to scuba dive with my family somewhere in Micronesia."

Diane explains that on Guam she spent magical days near or in the water. It's a strange and ironic dichotomy that as much as she fears swimming, she loves the ocean. "It's in my psyche. I remember being very little and part of the ritual in the Philippines [where her dad was born] is they teach the babies and little kids to swim by putting them on an adult back, and I remember—I was probably about four or five—my dad putting me on his back and us going into the ocean . . . It's such a safe-feeling memory."

But somehow, for her, swimming stops there. She was young and it's hard to remember, but she theorizes that her father became busy, and she was a girl, and girls weren't expected to do outdoorsy, adventurous things, even if the ocean did surround her home. There was no progression from that one moment clutching her father's shoulders, streaming through the warm, jade-colored water toward the reef, to learning to swim on her own. "I was always rewarded for my brains when I grew up. That was my area of expertise—smart girl, glasses, not athletic," Diane tells me. "That's the self-image I've had most of my adult life."

Ian says that he, also, used to have fears about swimming. "I really didn't like to put my face in the water," he tells her. It wasn't until his late twenties, when he realized he possessed almost all the ingredients to be great at triathlons—he raced all manner of bicycles, fast, and was a very strong runner—that the stakes became high enough for him to get into a pool and learn swimming for real. "And now I'm a really good swimmer," he says, nodding. He praises the reasons she came here to learn to swim, and adds that as she masters it, more reasons will crop up. "Swimming is one of those sports you can keep getting better at until you're ninety," he tells her. "It's so gentle on your body, it's a great workout, you can keep doing it."

Ian helps Diane fiddle with her goggles and the cap, getting the fit right. Focusing on the details is a welcome distraction, he seems to realize. When they finally walk to the pool edge and Diane stares down resolutely, a random onlooker would never know that she is nervous. I myself am aware of it only because we have talked beforehand. I also know that whatever Diane puts her mind to, she is likely to accomplish.

This is, after all, a woman with her own successful business as a consultant, who decided when she was almost fifty years old that it was time to get in shape. The previous ten years had been spent raising her first daughter, Coco, born premature with medical challenges. She and her husband threw themselves into life with a child who needed 24/7 supervision. After a decade, they adopted a second daughter, Lily Marie. "I did the math and I was going to be in my fifties when she was growing up. I wanted to be more active."

Most people would begin a gentle walking campaign, perhaps, or maybe join a gym and lift some baby weights.

Diane immediately started CrossFit, a discipline known for its no-wimps-here ethos and a regimen that includes pushing tires and climbing ropes. The community was supportive, so she suffered through the workouts; for Diane the satisfaction of surviving seemed to compensate for the lack of any real enjoyment. "CrossFit almost killed me," she confesses. When she had whupped herself enough and proved to herself that getting in shape was possible, Diane segued into other fitness pursuits, like Pilates and yoga. Soon she realized that the fitness routine that suited her best combined physical and energetic alignment. Swimming, part of her knew, might be ideal—especially if it allowed her to access her beloved ocean.

At some point Diane also decided that she needed to learn to camp. It was a skill that would allow her to participate in music festivals and spiritual retreats, not to mention keep up with adventurous Lily Marie. (Around this time, Lily wanted to skydive. Diane had to break it to her that it wasn't legal for a seven-year-old.) Again, Diane could have sussed out an outdoorsy friend, asked her for pointers on tent setup and camping food, maybe wrangled a weekend trip. Instead, she threw herself into a ten-week wilderness training course. This was the CrossFit version of learning how to get outside: on the first day they hiked fourteen miles. Diane was the only person who had never laced up a boot or worn a backpack. Fourteen miles! She'd only covered that in a car. She remembers she was miserable and lost a toenail. "I didn't know how to pee in the outdoors, so I didn't go to the bathroom the whole time." It was dark when she finally finished; she was the last person. She contemplated quitting the course altogether, but when an instructor told her not to judge the entire potential experience on one (brutal) hike, she agreed to persevere. In the end, the instructor was right—learning to equip herself for a trail walk and to cook and set up a tent outside was mind-blowing. ("But I could have done without the snow camping at thirty degrees below zero.") It opened up her life to what she calls "cultural adventuring." She could now dance to her heart's content at multiday outdoor music festivals; she watched a full solar eclipse from her campsite on an Oregon hill with people from all over the world. This was her jam, experiencing her life "culturally, spiritually, physically, and artistically . . . because I could sleep outdoors in a tent!"

Today the water is colder than Diane likes—she says she keeps her own tiny backyard pool, which has no deep end and can be traversed in just a few strokes, at ninety degrees. There is that moment of hesitation, but she jumps in. Ian tells her to go under all the way. She pauses, seems to be having a conversation in her brain (drown? drown?), then dunks herself.

Diane executes some awkward freestyle strokes, and Ian can see she isn't starting at zero, but yes, her movement is too frantic, too exhausting; it's no wonder she feels as if she can't stay afloat for long. Ian praises her, then explains that swimming is all about balance in the water—keeping the cap, bum, and heel level, thus minimizing drag. To that end, he tells her, they are going to concentrate on learning that symmetry today. Immediately, I am hopeful. "Balance," "symmetry"—these are words that Diane can relate to.

The first exercise is to push off the wall underwater, glide, then float upward, breaking the surface, head, buttocks, and heels at the same time. Ian demonstrates. Diane watches. When he rights himself and it's Diane's turn, she's nervous but trying to hide it. "Are people able to sink while they're alive?" she asks him, laughing a little, buying time. Then, as if she knows that deliberating another second will only make it harder, she quickly flips her body, presses her feet against the wall, and with a splash lurches forward, valiantly emulating what Ian has shown her.

The lesson proceeds from there—Ian explaining the exercise, Diane following suit a few times until she gets it right. She doesn't say she is scared, though she once sternly reminds him that she won't venture farther than the four-and-a-half-foot mark ("I'm not even five feet tall," she says), and I notice that Ian parks himself there, a silent reminder that he has heard her, that he won't let her drown. Later, Diane tells me she noticed this and it made her feel safer.

I love watching all this from the sidelines. I learned to swim when I was so young that I remember none of these principles. (Is my head in the right position when I swim? Turns out, no.) Also, I understand what it is taking for Diane to be on the surface, and then to put her face underwater, over and over again. She is scared, but she hasn't once said so. She has followed Ian's instructions fervently. She has even managed to look like she is enjoying herself.

When the lesson is over, Ian gives Diane homework— practice these skills for a few minutes every day. "Let's get together in two weeks," Ian says.

Diane tells me later that she loved her lesson. Ian was encouraging and laudatory when she needed it, but he corrected her and persisted until she performed a skill right. On the way home, she even bought herself her own goggles and swim cap. She would practice every day in her tiny shallow pool. In two weeks, she would be back.

I wait ten days before I contact her to find out how practice is going. Part of me knows that Diane is swimming diligently, overcoming her fears, pushing herself to meet her goals. This woman has snow-camped. She's pushed tires across gym floors. She's even recently returned from Japan and a pilgrimage along the ancient Kumano Kodo trail, which is forty-two miles long and takes five days to complete. Fear of water and a dislike of cold are no match for this Diane.

But another part of me thinks, Well, maybe not.

I email her to set up a quick chat. She doesn't get back to me right away. She's busy, of course, but it also makes me wonder. By the time we finally do talk, I am not surprised when she says she hasn't contacted Ian again and confesses that she hasn't been in the water at all. "Life and weather got in the way," Diane tells me sheepishly. There had been a cold spell, after all. She'd gotten busy. Hey, learning something new is hard to integrate. Especially when there is so much else going on.

. . .

Vijaya Srivastava, seventy-three, seems to be the type of person who would never learn to swim later in life. She has no previous experience with water or affinity with the ocean. Growing up in India in a conservative, protective family, swimming was "just not on their radar, or mine," she tells me. There was no access to swimming pools, and anyway, education was the priority. Beyond a few badminton games, Vijaya says, she didn't engage in any outdoor activities at all.

Vijaya married and moved with her husband to the United States in 1970. "I came to Buffalo—the weather was treacherous!" She'd never seen snow before, and when she did, she was mesmerized—"but you don't do anything with snow," she tells me. "You enjoy it from indoors."

Over the years she might walk a little with coworkers at lunch, but otherwise she did no exercise and felt no connection to nature. "I had a sedentary life," she confesses. Then, in 2014, after years of living in Detroit (more snow, she tells me), Vijaya and her husband moved to California to be closer to grandchildren. They settled into a condominium complex. There, right by the entrance gate, in plain view every time she made her way to her apartment, was a beautiful, sparkling, turquoise pool.

Proximity to a pool doesn't alone encourage swimming. It was only when, at sixty-eight, Vijaya told her doctor that she wanted to lose a few pounds perhaps, and her doctor added that her prediabetic numbers were creeping up, that things began to change. How about some exercise in that pool of yours? the doctor said. "I can't swim," Vijaya told her, thinking that would be that. The doctor responded, "Well, you can learn," and sent her home with a prescription: lessons.

At first Vijaya was sure that she was simply too old to learn something new. But she had been watching the children and adults play in the water since she'd moved here. It looked fun. It looked *really* fun. And Vijaya, who is quick to laugh and joke, is someone who likes fun. Why not, then? She approached her neighbor Preeti Dadlani, also sixty-eight; they had known each other about a year and were just getting to be good friends. "Do you want to learn how to swim?" Vijaya asked hopefully. Preeti said yes.

On the Nextdoor app they found a young swimming teacher—she was *tiny*, Vijaya tells me in a voice that narrates the moment in the horror movie when the door to the basement slowly opens. After all, how could a tiny girl save her and Preeti if they were to need help in deep water? But the teen assured them that she had lifeguard training, and that satisfied them both. She'd never trained any seniors, but that seemed fine, too. They approached this new, mysterious activity with just the right amount of naïveté and goodwill, it turns out. They began their lessons, one hour three times a week, in the condo pool.

Like Diane, Vijaya says she was "petrified to be in the water." But being accountable to her neighbor and friend meant that Vijaya turned up for the first lesson anyway. The pool itself seemed huge—twenty-two yards long, sloping gradually from three feet deep to eight feet deep at the far end. When the instructor asked what her swimming goals were, Vijaya exclaimed that all she wanted was to swim to the five-foot depth mark (she's five foot four) and back. But the young instructor—no pushover, it seems—told Vijaya to set her sights on the far end. "I promised I would. But I wasn't intending to keep that promise," Vijaya tells me now with an impish laugh.

The young instructor began that first day by teaching Vijaya how to put her face underwater (terrifying), hold her breath, blow bubbles. She also taught her how to float. "Floating I liked," Vijaya says. "It's relaxing. The problem was getting out of that position. I didn't know how to go from floating to back on my feet." It was like an astronaut working out weightlessness—there were so many of these small but vital kinetic conundrums in this confounding medium.

Vijaya prayed before each lesson. When I ask what exactly she prayed for, she confesses she asked God to bestow swimming effortlessly and immediately. A swimming miracle, in other words. She laughs about it now; that's not the way God, or swimming, works. She knew that, even at the time, but still, praying for a miracle was part of her swimming routine.

When the day came to first put her head underwater and actually swim, the prayers intensified. "It was exciting and exhilarating and all these emotions. But the dominating one was scariness. What if I drown?"

When I ask her why she persevered in the face of such fear, she shrugs, explaining that at an older age, there just aren't second chances. "It's a Cinderella moment. Once it strikes twelve, I'm DONE. I have to do it now." After a couple of weeks, dunking her face under wasn't scary anymore. Soon, she and Preeti were swimming the diagonal length of the pool in the shallow end. It was a short distance, and they could touch the bottom at any time. As they progressed, the instructor headed them in a different direction, toward the far end and that dreaded eight-foot depth marker.

Vijaya remembers when she finally faced her fingers-crossed promise. "One day my coach said, I think you're ready to go to the other end. But it sounded so scary. You're passing six feet, seven feet, eight feet. She said, I'll be next to you, I won't let you drown." Vijaya put it off, but soon got back into Cinderella mode, thinking, Well, if I don't swim those twenty-two yards now, I'll never do it.

"You have to take that leap. I had to trust her. But in my mind I said, let's just try to five feet [deep] and see how I feel." Once in the water, Vijaya swam a bit, then searched for the depth marker. "It said six feet! And I thought, now I couldn't turn around." She pauses and laughs. "For one, I didn't actually know how to turn around!" By this point, Vijaya was tired. She told this to her young coach, who seemed unconcerned and asked, "So what do you want to do?" Vijaya turned on her back to float and think. Feeling rested, she flipped on her stomach and swam a few more feet forward. "Then I flipped on my back and took a couple of breaths and let my limbs rest." Swimming, floating, swimming, floating. Suddenly the eight-foot depth marker loomed, right there. She reached for the pool edge, then grasped it, sputtering. She had made it. Neighbors rose from their sun chairs and their places in the hot tub, swept up in this slow-motion victory. They had watched Vijaya's progress for months; now she had done it. Vijaya remembers that she wanted to raise a hand in victory, or even acknowledge the surrounding support with a wave, but she didn't want to let go of the side, in case she sank to the bottom. Instead she listened while clutching the edge as her neighbors broke out into cheers and loud applause.

"It was one of the best feelings of my life, other than my grandchildren's births," she tells me.

She began to fall in love with the feeling of swimming. "I was just so taken over by it. The nights I couldn't sleep, I would emulate my swimming in bed, do my arms and kick. My husband would say, 'Hey, it's not the pool here,' and I would say, 'I'm just seeing how it feels on land.' It became my passion. I would watch every YouTube video I could find."

Her older age continued to shine as an advantage, not a hindrance. "The things that used to matter to me twenty years ago didn't matter anymore. I was no longer embarrassed . . . If I'm in a bathing suit and there's a bulge, so what. If I'm slower than others, who cares?!"

It helped that she began to see real change, not just in her swimming stroke, but in her body. All her markers started to get better—lipids, sugars, blood pressure. She lost weight. Her strength skyrocketed. She noticed she was no longer out of breath when she walked around her hilly California town. "They say I look stronger and I have better posture. I know I have more confidence. Because swimming isn't easy, so if I can learn something like that . . ."

. . .

Diane doesn't reach out for another lesson for a month and a half. When she does finally schedule, I am unable to attend, but Diane relays that it was great. She says that they worked on the freestyle technique, with Ian teaching her to roll with her core as she switched arms. Watching her hand slap the water at the entry, he suggested that she imagine instead putting mail in a slot, and also explained that she needed to get length in that arm reach. He described it as *"yearning* for length." Yearning. That she understood. She kicked forward to do the exercise, and for a fleeting moment, as her body stretched and twisted and she *yearned for length*, she realized what all the swimming fuss was about. Suddenly, her body felt *right* in the water. It was just a moment, she says now, but it was palpable, real. Then the moment was gone. But she was left with a hint of why swimming is lauded as so relaxing, so meditative.

Diane had most likely glimpsed "flow," a vaunted neurological state triggered by extreme concentration, whose hormonal side effects (dopamine, ocytocin, endorphins) gives it something akin to a religious feel. In her book *Why We Swim*, the author and swimmer (and my surfer friend) Bonnie Tsui describes in beautiful detail the reasons that swimming enables flow, citing scientists but also turning to poets for the right words, finally concluding after a dip in the river that "I am alone, but I don't feel lonely. To swim is to be a part of things." Indeed, flow feels all-encompassing, offering complete relaxation, a loss of time, and a feeling of synchronicity. Bonnie points out that "being in the zone" and "flow" are used interchangeably, but technically they differ—the former centering on heightened performance and the latter referring to a mental state. Factors like clear goals, immediate feedback, and a challenge-to-skills balance are foundational for the flow state, agrees Mihaly Csikszentmihalyi, the man who elevated the concept and coined the word; since then many have studied and written of the phenomenon, and expanded on the idea. There are as many as twenty-one triggers for flow, argues Steven Kotler in his book *The Art of Impossible*. These include novelty, unpredictability, and high stakes. "If you want more flow in your life, then build your life around these triggers," Kotler advises.

On some unconscious level, Diane has long been building her life around flow. She is a Pilates student, a yoga practitioner, a lover of dance and rhythm. A swimming lesson also holds the requisite triggers—clear goals, immediate feedback, and a skill component. Diane has now had this glimpse of flow in the pool, and I am eager to see whether she will increase her commitment to practice and lessons.

But then, nothing.

. . .

Vijaya welcomes me at the gate of her condo on a cold April morning wearing a red, calf-length insulated swim jacket, looking very much like the avid swimmer she has become. It's hard to square the woman who eyed the five-foot depth mark with fear while clinging to the side of the pool with the confident seventy-three-year-old in front of me. We chitchat as she expertly dons her cap and goggles and then moves to the side of the pool without hesitation. I fumble with my own new cap and goggles—I haven't swum in any directed way for at least six years—and follow Vijaya into the water.

Vijaya swims with joy. I'm not sure how to explain it. She is very earnest about her laps, stroking doggedly for each up-and-back lap before resting on the concrete lip, where-upon she flicks her wrist to check her watch for lengths and split times. Yet she is not fixated on the metrics. She is enchanted also by the mere movement of wind-milling arms, kicking feet, and shifting hips, thrilled with the effort, smiling and unhurried in her rest. Her stroke is not exactly elegant (early on her husband exclaimed how amazing it was that she could swim mostly with one arm, she tells me) but it is majestic in its care and fervor. I rest with her, and we talk.

It becomes clear that unlike Diane, Vijaya and Preeti swam often outside of the lessons, practicing what they'd learned. They even filmed themselves with their phones and peered at the footage for insight into their strokes and breathing. Sometimes at the end of a swim session, Vijaya tells me, they would pull themselves up the ladder flipping their hair, swinging a hip, emulating the actress Bo Derek emerging from the pool in the iconic movie *10*. They routinely found this hysterical, sixty-eight-year-olds likening themselves to a young sex symbol and bombshell. Sure, this mimicry was for the sheer absurdity and fun of it, and Vijaya relays it even now with a laugh. But I can't help thinking that this feigned pageantry also expresses their own newfound empowerment, physical health, and pride.

Vijaya's swimming success led to other ventures. She began to walk the hills behind her home. "I thought, if I can swim, I can certainly do that." Then came yoga, something that had always intrigued her; at one of our pool-edge pit stops, she demonstrates yogic breathing, huffing out loudly, intentionally bobbing her diaphragm. "This massages the organs," she tells me.

At another pit stop, Vijaya warns me kindly that since I am not in swim shape, I might want to stop soon; I don't want to be too sore tomorrow, do I? "Good sore," she reminds me. "Not bad sore." I agree, and head to the shallow end to exit. I've been swimming since I was four years old, but now I'm shimmying from the water well before my seventy-three-year-old friend, who will complete four more laps (eight more pool lengths) while I shower and then write down some notes.

Sometime later, I check back in with Diane. Over a period of months, she has managed three lessons and six to seven practices in her pool. When I phone her to debrief, she is candid. "The deep end, this is where I have always stopped my lessons . . . I want to figure out a different way so I don't repeat that." What will that different way be? Will she get over this hump? It is unclear.

I have to admit it: I am a little disappointed. Part of me was certain that aging brought an extra urgency, and surely this would propel us through the sticking points. Wasn't Vijaya's Cinderella moment, where the clock is about to strike twelve on all of us, a powerful incentive? But perhaps success is not to be measured by the goal one sets out to accomplish. There can be interim successes that are less obvious but perhaps even more significant. Diane got herself to the pool, and she gamely completed three lessons. She faced her phobias and did more than she expected. "Experientially, I was able to see that when the skills start coming, the fear goes," she tells me. It isn't about focusing on the psychological, she sees, it is about beefing up the skill set, so that swimming becomes comfortable, not exhausting. But she just hasn't been able to put in the time to reach that pivotal moment where her skill outmatches her trepidation. The truth is, Diane has a full life as a successful businesswoman, involved mother, loving wife, dancer at music festivals, hiker of trails. She doesn't actually need to learn to swim to the deep end in order to find fulfillment. Ultimately, not every outdoor activity is right for everyone. We try, and in the trying there are glimpses of important things, like novelty, challenge, courage, even triumph, even if not actually the ultimate win. At this point, really, the better question is not *will Diane learn to swim,* but *does it really matter?*

When I ask Vijaya the secret to her swimming success, she points first and foremost to the buddy system. Enlisting her friend to swim had been pivotal. "You motivate each other. Certain mornings, I would say, 'I don't feel like swimming,' and my friend would say, 'Just come down for twenty minutes.' I would think, if I don't go she won't, so . . ." She went. Always.

I ask her if she will be taking the next pelagic step—to open-water swimming. She shakes her head. The visibility in the bay is nil (which I know well), the water cold. "I like seeing the bottom," she says. "And I hear you get seaweed stuck on you!" That doesn't mean she doesn't have more swimming goals. She'd like to be able to get into the water from the side of the pool, instead of walking down steps or a ladder. She explains how she recently tried to dive in from a sitting position—rolling toward the water with her arms forward—but she held her head too high. "It was so much pain!" she exclaims now, describing what sounds to me like a face belly flop. She isn't giving up, though. If a dive doesn't work, perhaps she'll learn to jump in instead. She'd also like to become better at treading water—something she knows how to do but hasn't mastered yet (instead she uses the floating-on-the-back method). Finally, she wants to be able to swim to the bottom of the pool, as the kids do. She once lost a bracelet while swimming, and it was her grandchildren who ultimately retrieved it. "I've tried, but I just float back up when I get near the bottom," she says. I love hearing about all these goals, and I imagine her in the near future, kicking hard toward the blue tiled floor, smile wide, both ears perked to the imaginary clock about to strike twelve, one arm outstretched, reaching, reaching for the bangle of gold.

9

Find Your Way

You must never stop being whimsical. And you must not,
ever, give anyone else responsibility for your life.

—MARY OLIVER, POET

On my drive to Briones Regional Park today, I follow the gentle urging of my GPS. *Turn right in five hundred feet*, intones the voice, resembling something between high school principal and friendly phone scammer. *Take the left fork.* I am obedient; this outsourcing to technology allows me to forgo logistics and instead throw appreciative glances at the golden hills and soaring hawks outside my car window. Even as I see the landscape, though, my sense of where I actually am is nil. North or south? In relation to my hometown of San Francisco? No idea.

This is an irony that resonates, since I am about to meet someone who spends a lot of her life knowing exactly where she resides in a given landscape. Penny DeMoss is an avid participant (and frequent winner) in the sport of orienteering, which she defines for me as "off-trail running with a map and compass." I soon learn that this is a vast understatement: for Penny, orienteering is actually a full-tilt dash across dastardly terrain, often for upward of eight miles, to various checkpoints that lie behind stones and through brambles and up hills, all the while knowing exactly where north is, and her corresponding location on the paper map she holds in her hand.

Luckily for me, Penny has kindly agreed to walk, not run, the orienteering course that lies ahead, one that she herself set up for this occasion. It helps that she recently broke her foot while negotiating a steep downhill during a race (her sneaker caught a protruding root; her body continued forward but her foot did not.) Her injury is not at all evident when I meet her. Neither is her age; with long brown hair that falls mid-back, and a lithe but sturdy figure, Penny doesn't look like your average white, American, seventy-two-year old female. I also know that her husband has recently finished the last of his forty-five radiation sessions, but she gives me her full attention despite this distraction and is soon handing me a map and explaining its keys and features.

I'm interested in orienteering as an outdoor activity for the simple reason that I am often lost. Even in the city I have lived in for almost forty years, I get turned around, and can walk blocks before realizing I am heading in the wrong direction. Some people I know are always oriented to the cardinal points;

not me. This seemed just an inconvenient quirk until I began to hear that navigation was inextricably linked to memory, and therefore that recent technologies meant to ease our travel—GPS, most notably—might be doing more harm than good. The more we orient ourselves in unfamiliar space by relying on these aids, research suggests, the more some important parts of our brain might begin to fail.

This freaked me out. I didn't want to lose my memory. I must get better, I told myself, at directional comprehension. I took to carrying a compass and testing myself by guessing my direction at random times, then checking it against the bobbling red needle, aghast at how wrong I was. I eschewed GPS and bought paper maps, annoying my wife constantly by insisting, before we left on a trip, on squinting at the tiny index of street names, then running my fingers along the grid to locate our endpoint, while her smartphone shook out a blue line in milliseconds, ready to point the way. I relearned how to awkwardly unfurl these maps, then karate-chop the seams to a semi-manageable size and lay them on the passenger seat, leaning over now and then to check my progress as I drove. More than once I took wrong turns on small country roads. I overshot necessary highway exits. My car wandered onto the rumble strips as I tried to side-eye the tiny lines and numbers. Gradually, under duress from the people around me, I succumbed and went back (with some relief, I admit) to the ease of GPS. But I remained worried about my spatial confusion, and curious whether the sport of orienteering would be a safer and more efficient way to stave off what turns out to be one of our biggest fears as we age—memory loss and brain disease.

Today, Penny looks like the fit, capable trail runner she is. I sport a compass hanging around my neck, a baseball cap over a ponytail, a vest over a long-sleeve shirt, and an industrial-size fanny pack, looking much like a parody from a *Saturday Night Live* skit. The picture is complete when I bend to tuck my socks into my long pants (ticks?); Penny says it isn't necessary, and do I want to take the compass from my neck to avoid continually throttling myself whenever it's in use?

The first order of business after sunscreen is applied and hat brims settled is straightforward: find north. No fancy numbered degrees, no east, west, south. Just north. Not even true north, just magnetic north. (Magnetic north migrates, and most paper maps are in true north, so you have to do math that accounts for the "variation" in your geographic area that year. Variation is also speeding up—since 2020 it has increased to, on average, a whopping twenty-seven miles annually, as compared to an average of nine miles in previous decades. This is due, scientists think, to sudden shifts in earth's molten core.) My compass in hand, I watch the red arrow spin, bobble, then calm. "North!" I exclaim excitedly, while pointing to my right in triumph.

Penny instructs me to match this IRL magnetic north to my magnetic north map, which I also think I quickly master, until she gently suggests that the map may be upside down (yes). Fully oriented now, we head on a well-trod path toward the start. Official starts during competition are often as much as a mile away from the place where you assemble; once there, you turn over the map, suss out its required checkpoints, and begin. "It's you and the map against the clock," Penny says.

And against the terrain. Once the first checkpoint is located on the map, the participant is faced with a dilemma: what is the fastest way to reach it? Could it simply be the shortest—which often means bushwhacking—or would it be smarter to divert to the longer but easier route—less steep, smoother, simpler? The brain workout is palpable as I puzzle over what is also a familiar metaphor—a well-trod life path, or the dazzling leap into wild underbrush? In orienteering, perhaps as in life, the answers come after a quick analysis of both the topography and one's own skill. Penny says that she almost always runs the shortest route, knowing that she can handle pretty much any terrain (except: "I won't go through poison oak.") Which is why we quickly leave the asphalt behind and cut across a rutted field to a fence line (a "catching feature," she explains), me stumbling frequently, and why once the beep of her receiver tells us we've found the first checkpoint, she points straight across a field of high this-tles to the hill beyond and declares that we'll reach the second checkpoint that way. (Today we are prompted by electronic waypoints that Penny has preset on a virtual map of our real terrain, but much of orienteering uses real check-points into which one inserts a reader to indicate you were there.)

I am reminded that Penny grew up with many waypoints already placed at difficult vantages. When she was a girl, for instance, it was unthinkable for her to run any distance lest, as many athletic coaches at the time warned, her uterus and ovaries promptly fell out. As a young teen she tried out for the all-boys cross-country team anyway, because there was no option at the time for girls. But she was cut—not because she was too slow, but because she was too fast. "The coach said, go home and stop showing off," she tells me. Years passed, and then she saw Frank Shorter win the 1972 Olympic marathon. She had no idea that people ran that far, and, energized, she began to train again, almost always on her own. It was so unusual to see a woman running that she was once stopped by cops who thought she must be fleeing someone. Undeterred, she entered local races in the San Francisco Bay Area, like the fabled Dipsea and the Bay to Breakers, and finally marathons, and her success in these competitions landed her on the cover of *Runner's World* twice, in 1977 and 1978. During those years she also held down a job as staff artist for a big magazine, married a fellow marathoner, became a stepmom, chaired committees that organized women's running events, and ran more than one hundred miles a week. Yet she seemed unfazed by the overall workload, telling *Runner's World* that "there is nothing mystical or psychological about my morning runs. They wake me up and get me going for the day."

The thistles, head high and flowering purple, join with towering yellow mustard plants, so that the effect is of pushing through a Van Gogh painting. I've abandoned the map and am instead simply following Penny, though quickly she becomes just parts of herself amid the colors—a brown ponytail, a pale white nose, a bright green baseball cap, then she disappears completely. The thistles nip and bite. It's not hot out, but I am sweating anyway. "You'd be running through this?" I yell forward to her, as I stumble for the umpteenth time, and her disembodied voice shouts back, "Yes!" My mind lights on horror movies and protagonists who push frantically through cornstalks, but the day is too beautiful to stay there long, and instead I begin to admire the stalwart resistance of nature, her resolute pricks, her face slaps of purple and yellow. Not to mention the stalwart attributes of the orienteer ahead of me, who breaks thistle trail with nary a tiny *Ow* to indicate discomfort. Finally, we emerge onto a wide footpath, me blinking at the scratches on my hand and exuberant to have made it through, Penny already looking skyward at the rising golden hill and the tree halfway up its flank.

Penny has volunteered since 2007 with a wildlife rehabilitation organization, and her concern for helpless creatures may help explain her patience with a newbie orienteer like me. At any given moment Penny's house is likely to have at least a few furry animals scratching around in her artist-studio-turned-nursery. Her specialty, she tells me, is wood rats and bunnies, with an expertise in infant wood rats. Baby wood rats are notoriously hard to raise, needing to be fed every few hours, using tiny syringes. ("People from all over the United States call me," she says in a matter-of-fact voice.) This is why these days Penny limits herself to orienteering competitions she can travel to and complete in a certain time, depending on the needs of the orphans in her care. On fostering and its confines, she admits, "Sometimes I rue the day I started."

My map has lost its north orientation during the bush-whack, so Penny waits for me to realign. I glance from map to terrain and back again, feeling the familiar confusion. Then I take a breath and knuckle down to the task. After a moment, the landscape and the map seem to merge just enough, and I declare that the next checkpoint is—finger points—*somewhere near that tree, because*—swing the finger back to the map and run it along the topo lines—*of that indent, valley, slope?* I struggle for the word. It's a reentrant, Penny tells me, and nods sagely. Turns out, there are terms of art for all the various nooks and crannies of a landscape—ditch, water feature, seasonal drainages, spur, contour—offering me a more clinical but no less interesting way to understand and appreciate the landscape.

I begin the mental calculation again—path of least resistance, or most direct route? I peer hopefully at the trail we stand on, represented on the map by long dotted black lines ("large foot path," explains the map key). If I'm reading the contour lines right—Penny helps me here—it gains altitude slowly as it winds around the hill; this we could walk without difficulty for as long as possible before diverting back into the high grass and deep ruts of the reentrant. I think to myself how nice the smooth, unencumbered surface would be. And what a fine example of taking the longer route but getting to the checkpoint faster because of its ease.

I stare longingly to the flat trail, then swing my gaze back.

"Straight up?" I say.

"Definitely," Penny answers.

This type of hardiness is embedded in the sport, which began in the late 1800s as a way for the Swedish military to train their men in overland navigation, then morphed into a competitive sport as these soldiers took up civilian life. It remains highly popular in all the Scandinavian countries, as well as the rest of Europe and Britain, where more than thirty years ago a forty-year-old Penny learned the sport. There, "you can race two to three times a week." But here in the United States, for reasons that baffle Penny, orienteering remains obscure. "You're lucky to do it twice a month here," she says. I wonder if the idea of charging through thickets and thorns just doesn't appeal, given that most Americans expect well-maintained, clearly marked trails in their outdoor experiences. Penny isn't sure, but adds that she once took her best friend, also a very fast and avid trail runner, on a course. She was sure he would fall in love immediately, as she had. Instead, he hated it. "You call this fun?" he asked her, scraped and sweating and struggling to keep up.

The tree is reached and the receiver in Penny's hand beeps. Panting, I peer at the map for Checkpoint 3. (Penny reminds me that if this were a real race, she'd be planning her next route while still running.) I show her the two possibilities, and she asks me which one I want. "The one you would take in a race," I say with bravado.

Once again we find ourselves eschewing the wide path below and instead clinging to the side of a hill, making our way along its steep flank, keeping an eye on the point ahead that promises to reveal the checkpoint. There is no elevation gain, but I'm jerking around to stay upright, the crumbling edge giving me only enough room to place one foot in front of the other. Even at this careful pace, I slip and stumble and windmill my arms like one of those weird inflatable "air dancers" in front of retail stores. "You'd be running right now?" I ask, amazed (yes).

The next few checkpoints proceed in similar fashion: an assured march by Penny, much flailing and tripping by me. In fact, Penny knows the almost-exact number of running steps (she is rusty on the walking steps) it takes her to go a kilometer, which she then varies slightly with each race terrain ("it's forty-five left foot strides every one hundred meters, but if it's uphill it's fifty—or even sixty strides, if it's really steep"). This allows her to run all out while counting, then to stop in front of the right tree or stone or ditch behind which her checkpoint lurks. My own stride seems to have no rhyme or reason. It is sometimes assured ("large foot path") but mostly faltering ("dense undergrowth," "indistinct path"). I do have the wherewithal to exclaim often at the stunning views from each spur, the vistas from every reentrant. Each time, Penny seemed a little startled, and once I see her look around as if to check. It's not that nature doesn't speak to her, it is just saying vastly different things to her than to me. She definitely loves and cares for wildlife. But while she is racing, at least, nature is an anvil on which her mind and body are forged into harder steel, not softened into awe and wonder. She loves orienteering not for the reasons I would love it (the hard-won beauty) but, she tells me, because it is "running and thinking."

"At the heart of successful navigation," writes M. R. O'Connor in her book *Wayfinding: The Science and Mystery of How Humans Navigate the World*, "is a capacity to record the past, attend to the present and imagine the future—a goal or place we'd like to reach." This is the "thinking" that Penny is alluding to—the way the brain has to really click and whir to make sense of all the temporal and spatial cues, along with historical information about her abilities on this particular terrain and the math of her running speed, to finally conclude, *go there.* O'Connor explains that navigation is roughly divided into two different strategies—the "egocentric," as researchers call it, described as "rely[ing] on the traveler's point of view and relationship to objects around them," and the "allocentric," which means navigating using a mental bird's-eye view of the landscape, akin to opening up an atlas in your brain and staring at Siberia. We often shift between the two perspectives, O'Connor says.

Memory champions who go as far back as ancient Greece and Rome knew on an intuitive level that navigation and memory were linked. To take advantage of this they developed the method of loci, where one is able to recite the number pi, say, by associating each digit with a physical place. A "memory palace"—often the blueprint of a familiar location—is constructed in the mind, which is then wandered through. This door, that painting on the wall, the open window, are all subscribed a successive piece of information for retrieval as the brain saunters by. Alight on the first step of a staircase: *1*. Pass the ornate finial at the top: *4*. (In 2015, Rajveer Meena from India recited pi to the seventy-thousandth decimal point from memory, a feat that took a little over nine hours. If he used the method of loci, the place he wandered through must have been gigantic.)

Both memory and navigation are processed in the hippocampus, so injury there means you not only lose your capacity to find your way, but also much of your ability to consolidate enough memories to keep together an ongoing sense of self. The navigation your hippocampus excels at, then, is not just one of finding your location on a landscape. The hippocampus is also continually mooring your place in the world, psychologically and intellectually. In other words, this ability to make mental maps of geographical places accounts also for our skill at mental maps of abstract ideas, and of selfhood. O'Connor cites neuroscientist Howard Eichenbaum, whose research credits the hippocampus for "mapping and sequencing multidimensional aspects of our experience in addition to space, from time itself to social relationships to music."

My own hippocampus is clanking away. I try to make sense of the map and the terrain to untangle a route to Checkpoint 7. As I look at where we've been, and place us on the paper, I feel both the egocentric and the allocentric kicking in.

"What do you see?" Penny prompts.

"A water feature . . ." There is a grinding of gears in my brain.

Penny waits, then adds helpfully, "Near a lone tree, see?" She points at the map. "That will tip us off where to go in. When we go farther up there will be a small copse"—she points again—"and a larger copse, then a junction."

"I see it!" I exclaim, as if finally deciphering an ancient scroll.

The concrete link between memory and navigation is best seen in London taxi drivers, who have to pass a test that requires them to remember and navigate to more than twenty-five thousand streets and thousands of landmarks; MRI scans showed that their posterior hippocampi were considerably bigger than average; the more time they had logged as cabbies, the bigger the region. This is exciting, and heartening, because it implies that our memory and navigational skills can improve. Another study found that older volunteers who navigated using virtual reality showed marked long-term memory improvement compared to a control group. Your memory can get better, maybe even much better, by beefing up your spatial orientation skills, these studies say.

Unfortunately, this is not yet evident with me, since as we near the last checkpoint I again have trouble aligning to north. I am twisting my own body in circles to chase the red compass arrow, instead of just turning the map in my hands. Penny waits patiently. This has been an easy jaunt for her, and perhaps a difficult reminder that she can't yet push her foot injury (for a few of the checkpoints, Penny took stock of both my dishevelment and the thistle patch ahead, and offered to call it good if I simply pointed to where the checkpoint would be). Until baby wood rats got in the way, Penny routinely ran the longer, ten-to-fifteen-kilometer orienteering races. Once she and her husband, Harold, teamed up for a course that lasted over eight hours, which they won, trouncing much younger racers. Harold was faster than she for the first five years, she tells me, but then she surpassed him. Her highest placement at the annual world championships, up against the demigods of Scandinavia? Tenth, an impressive ranking, especially for an American; we are considered the Jamaican bobsledders of the sport, obscure and underfunded. So I am curious: As she has aged, has she become less competitive? Less steely? Has she found the grace in other aspects of the sport?

"No," she says bluntly. If she doesn't do well in a race, she "still get[s] really annoyed. If you blow one, you remember." For the past few years, her times have ebbed ("it came on very sudden, in my mid-to-late sixties—I was still pretty fast until then"). This slower pace does mean she tends to make fewer navigational mistakes; when she was younger, it was easy to miss checkpoints because "we would outrun our mental capabilities." That's good, I point out, and she tentatively agrees. When I ask how she handles the decline overall, she says judicially and after a pause, "I don't embrace it."

Penny recently released her latest wood rat. She prepared her by giving her sticks every night, with which the wood rat made her "midden." Penny then placed this nest and the wood rat into a box, which was slatted to allow exit and return, but also deterred any potential predator animals. "I take her to the woods, leave her there," Penny tells me, "and cry all the way back in the car." Her sudden vulnerability, after her no-nonsense, impervious-to-prickers-and-steep-hills attitude, takes me by surprise. It makes me realize that this process of rearing and then releasing demands toughness, a layer of crust over a soft heart, and it is that layer of crust that she also calls on in an orienteering race.

The wood rat crate is placed in the same area where all the other wood rats have been released over the years, so they find each other, Penny explains. Slowly and safely the wood rat becomes comfortable with her environment; soon she encounters her peers (or so Penny hopes) and transfers her midden, leaving her box behind. Eventually, Penny walks back and retrieves the crate. Each time, "the sticks are all gone," indicating success. As she talks, I imagine a tiny village of wood rats who emerge from behind tree stumps and bushes to love-bomb Penny when she next hikes in. I almost blurt out this vision, but think Penny would find it silly, and I don't want to betray that I sometimes wander from magnetic north into such flights of fancy.

Orienteering is a full-body experience, and as we tromp through a field trying to find the last point, I wipe the sweat from my brow, pick off foxtails (when I initially asked Penny what I should wear for our orienteering lesson, she said, "Socks you can throw away"), and realize I'm tired. But this bushwhacking is an integral part of the charm (and Penny assures me that novice orienteering races keep participants on easier terrain). There is also an added benefit, beyond the obvious ones of cardiac and muscular health. Studies show that physical interaction while trying to problem-solve improves results. Psychology professors Frédéric Vallée-Tourangeau and Gaelle Vallée-Tourangeau found that those who tackle an intellectual conundrum, and who interacted on multiple sensory levels with it (writing it down, for instance, or making three-dimensional models), did statistically better than those who reasoned and calculated in their heads. The two researchers conclude that "thinking with your brain alone—like a computer does—is not equivalent to thinking with your brain, your eyes, and your hands." Orienteering, which I can attest calls upon your body in both taxing and exhilarating ways, takes this idea of physical interaction in problem solving to new heights. Could it be that walking in difficult terrain while sweating, panting, and being stuck by thistles may be one of the most efficient ways to grow my navigation skills, and with them my memory?

There is no confetti or applause to indicate that the last checkpoint has been found, just the same high-pitched beep, but I feel as if I've been handed a gold trophy anyway. As we head back to the car on the large footpath we entered on, I wonder to myself why more doctors don't prescribe orienteering to help the aging brain as well as the aging body.

Suddenly—it only takes that moment of distraction—the landscape is strange and unfamiliar. I slow and gaze around, but say nothing to Penny. Then I shift the paper, pinpoint north beckoning at my shoulder, and, just like that, I am found.

HEART

10

Accept Loss

Cure yourself with the light of the sun and the rays of the moon
With the sound of the river and the waterfall
With the swaying of the sea and the fluttering of birds . . .

—MARIA SABINA, MAZATECA SHAMAN
AND POET (1894–1985)

I llona Aguayo doesn't want to be in her house these days. She would much rather unlock her small plastic kayak from its rack, push it off the dock, maneuver herself expertly onto its seat, and head out into the winding waterways of this Southern California marina. Fog, rain, wind, sun—the weather doesn't matter. She wants only to be outside, where she can gaze at birds, the pattern water makes in sunlight, the seal that pokes his head up to stare. Illona, a former high school teacher, is an artist, so she looks with the eye of a disciplined painter, searching for line, shape, and inspiration. But these days it's also something else. Being outside is a way to focus and to distract herself. When she's in nature, she tells me, she can get lost in the beauty around her. "Instead of thinking what I'm usually thinking. Which is about losing Louie."

Louie is Illona's husband, who died only seven months earlier. I am right now paddling the kayak that he would normally be sitting in. As I clumsily drop myself onto its bright yellow top, then whack a little at the water to steady myself, I hope I am worthy of this morning's journey. I'm not the first person to sit here since Louie's death; if someone wants to accompany her, Illona is happy to offer up the extra boat. But it's often hard to find women her age to paddle with, and anyway she's just as comfortable going alone. No matter what, she hits the water three times a week, for what she calls her spiritual rejuvenation, the kayaks as a perfect liturgy. The moment is at once unassuming—two Californians out for a morning paddle—and yet also sacred. I dip my paddle with care and the stained glass water shimmers with the color of our kayaks. Ahead is the cawing choir of seagulls, and a cathedral ceiling of morning fog.

Illona looks much younger than her almost-seventy years, with a long history of fitness behind her—she was an accomplished bodybuilder at one point, she ran marathons, and she even applied to be a Los Angeles police officer back in the early 1980s, where she was number one in her academy class (that iconic six-foot wall you have to climb over? It was a cinch, she tells me), a job she didn't accept after her then-husband said he would be too worried about her. Her kayaks are simple affairs—stubby at nine feet long, stable at almost three feet wide, and molded from plastic. The kayaker then perches on the hardy outer shell, something made a little more comfortable by an attachable seat pad (always wet from the water that seeps through its self-bailing holes), but otherwise the boat resembles nothing so much as a log with a few hydrodynamic angles. The paddles are simple, too—just oar shapes on each end of a plastic tube; you alternately dip each side into the water, pull a little, and repeat. I love sit-on-tops, as these craft are affectionately called, for their ease of use, their safety, and their affordability. They track just fine. They don't sink. They rarely tip. They weather all manner of scratches and gashes with aplomb—I once saw a sit-on-top just ten minutes after it had been paddled into waters recently chummed by a fishing boat, an inexplicably dumb move by its owner. Quickly a great white shark feeding on the fish carcasses mistook the bright yellow plastic boat for something edible and took a bite. The teeth marks were evident, but the kayak remained afloat and ready for a paddle—not so the terrified human atop it, who was knocked overboard. If you do happen to get bucked off, like this poor guy, you simply haul yourself back on without much ado (adrenaline makes it especially easy, and the shark lost interest, too)—there is no hull to fill with water, and the boat floats upside down as well as right side up. For all these reasons, sit-on-tops are used by both beginners and the experienced. It is an egalitarian kayak for those without snobbery, perhaps a tendency to lapses in judgment, and a tolerance for a wet butt.

This is not a wilderness expedition; around us squat fishing vessels are tied up next to gleaming yachts (one is actually painted gold); Zodiacs bump up to sailboats. But there are few humans about, and the pelicans swoop, and it smells like the sea. The fog has yet to clear, and ground mist shrouds the embankment, turning it Amazonian. It blurs our edges and adds a hush, but we still easily spot the first seals of the day, sprawled on an empty dock, woven together like puppies, some squirming to get comfortable under the formidable weight of another, but mostly resting. Illona and I float and watch. Now and then one seal raises her head to yap angrily or maybe just bark a thought—it's hard to tell what is idle conversation and what is territorial warning, and this adds to the feeling that, despite the large boats, and the very fancy houses lining the water, Illona and I are not completely in civilization.

Illona kayaks her sit-on-top the way I do—a few strokes, and then a pause to talk in her thick New Jersey accent (think *The Sopranos*, but then add a paddle jacket and a stylish haircut of bangs and long, layered gray hair), telling me the history of the marina or answering a question about her past. Today I am very interested in how being outdoors is helping her through one of the most dreaded, and perhaps most common, parts of the aging process—the death of a loved one.

My own experience is limited. I did, however, lose my father when I was in my early forties, and he seventy-eight. He suffered from emphysema and had moved in his final years to live near me. I saw him almost every day. It was in many ways a beautiful time, for which I was totally unprepared, and I spent way too much of it fussing about cleaning his house or distracted by my own life while in his company. But on the days I presented my better self, we spent hours watching *Antiques Roadshow*, or marveling at the TV psychic John Edwards, who routinely squinted at an audience member and then pronounced that she had once had a dog and should resolve those issues with her boss. We dined at a local greasy spoon many mornings and ate simple dinners of sandwiches and chocolate. My father rarely felt specific pain, but there must have been a lot of anxiety; he told me once how much he missed the feeling that came with taking a deep breath (emphysema makes it difficult to fully expel air, so that some always remains and inhibits new oxygen intake). Despite my inevitable shortcomings as a caretaker, when he lapsed into a coma I had no regrets (those would come later as I thought about how much more patient I could have been, more attentive). It was no coincidence, too, what happened after twenty-four hours of standing vigil. My father had been breathing raggedly for hours, far past what the doctors and nurses expected after oxygen was removed. My twin, exhausted, stepped out for twenty minutes to run an errand, leaving me alone with him, and it was at that time that my father chose to depart. I was reading a mindless, distracting *People* magazine supplied by the hospital, I remember, and suddenly jerked my head up. What made me do it is unclear, but later I wondered if my father had tapped me on the shoulder to say goodbye. It was just me and him at the end, and that seemed right, an acknowledgment of those past few years. I walked the three steps to his bed and wept onto his silent chest.

The loss of a partner, though, is different from the loss of a parent. And for Illona, it happened way too early. Illona is sixty-eight. Louie had been sixty-one. She'd had to watch him deteriorate for a year, the restrictions of the pandemic making a lonely process at home even more difficult, with all the mundane, heartrending tasks of caretaking executed without help even at the very end. Then there were decisions to make. There were no kids. They owned a house. They even had an RV (Illona has visited almost every national park, with four to go). They'd hiked, ridden motorcycles, kayaked together. But it was Louie who had done most of the maintaining, fixing, planning—for instance, it was he who loaded up these very kayaks in the truck each time, ferried them to the marina, unloaded them.

"Initially I thought, What do I do? Sell all this stuff?" But Illona loved the outdoors. How could she give it up? Before her marriage she'd been very independent—she had ridden her Harley motorcycle solo across much of Europe, camping all the way, for goodness' sake. And just because a few guys told her it was impossible, she'd driven a simple 150cc motor-cycle—the equivalent of a scooter, according to them—from New Jersey to Colorado, proving them wrong. (She makes sure I realize that, even back then, when she was young, it wasn't easy. "It's not that I wasn't afraid. I was always afraid. I just overcame it.") Not to mention all those decades she'd taught art to that most fearsome of audiences, high school teenagers. "I thought, Wait a minute, you used to do all this on your own." She was determined to overcome her trepidations.

When I ask her what those trepidations are, specifically, she laughs. "I'd never driven a twenty-seven-foot RV!" And it wasn't just the driving; what about once she had driven to the trailhead? "It's scary to hike alone because there are rattlesnakes and bobcats." But she was no pushover. She decided she could do it; she just needed to be prepared.

But how best to prepare? How does a sixty-eight-year-old widow take the first necessary steps to renewed independence? With instructional videos on YouTube, of course. "There are so many good videos out there," she tells me. "I think it's amazing what we can learn with it. Sometimes I think I've invented something, and I YouTube it, and nope, someone has thought of it first."

Take the kayaks. She rented a slip, then typed "kayak racks" into the search bar, bought one, and assembled it dockside, wielding a screwdriver while peering at an instructional video on her phone. Voilà! Now there was no need to load the boats from home onto the truck each time—she could just keep them at the marina. She would drag the lower kayak off its rack, pull it along the dock the few short feet to the water's edge, then push it in from there; if the second kayak on the upper rack was needed, too, it could be lifted with the friend who has come to use it. Sounds simple, but it took some thinking through, and initiative. And YouTube.

It is obvious to me that what Illona has done is a feat. It's so difficult to overcome the anxieties, the inertia, the many years of depending on someone else, not to mention the overwhelming grief. Any quest for renewed independence is also the ultimate admission that Louie is no longer there taking care of things. It must hurt extra, that at every juncture where she succeeds, there is the gaping hole of Louie. But she waves me off when I say this. "I always think about him anyway," she tells me.

It would be tempting to try to fit Illona's experience, and specifically her integration of the outdoors, into the Kübler-Ross Five Stages of Grief and come up with a prescription. But it is increasingly clear that mourning, much like the gifts of the outdoors itself, is not easily quantifiable. In her 1999 book, *Ambiguous Loss: Learning to Live with Unresolved Grief*, the therapist and professor Pauline Boss wholeheartedly rejects the Kübler-Ross paradigm, frowning at its linear trajectory, clearly defined categories, and eventual promise of sadness overcome. Bereavement, she counters, conjures a mishmash of emotions not easily partitioned, nor does that grief necessarily have an endpoint. It clings to us in differing ways with varying intensities, perhaps forever. This is difficult for Americans, Boss says, steeped as we are in the rhetoric that hard work leads to chosen outcomes we can readily control.

When Louie died, there were the difficult days and then the really bad days, Illona tells me. "The bad days were triggered by a piece of mail, like by the insurance company questioning the process, did he really need a stent? Those are the things that would bring me crashing down. But I realized, you have a choice. You could hide under the covers, or you could go out and kayak."

We twist and turn through the marina's waters as we talk; repeatedly I lose my bearings (surprise). I have no idea which way the ocean is, but Illona always does, pointing her paddle when I ask. Every now and then a duck surfaces and jerks her head toward us. One by one, each clocks our languid forward motion, quickly rules out predator behavior, and turns back to the bugs in the water. These small moments keep repeating—a duck here, a pelican there, a seal slapping the water. It is perhaps the familiarity of the marina, coupled with the tiny surprises, that persuades Illona to come back over and over and over, and to keep slowly healing.

It wasn't long after Louie's death that Illona decided she would take a trip, and she would do it in the RV. Sure, she really didn't know the first thing about any of it, except how to cook dinner, which had been her contribution during their travels. But this would be a way to show herself that despite the loss of a beloved adventure companion, there was still her independent self to call upon. Also, she wanted—no, *needed*—to access the wilderness. It calmed and inspired her in the best of times. Now, during these days of grief and mourning, she needed it even more.

The RV was intimidating, she tells me, no doubt about it. But "everything is a state of mind. If you're already thinking negatively about something, it's not going to be good. If you imagine yourself able to do it, it changes everything. You can adapt to anything. You just have to be willing." Illona was willing. She knuckled down, knowing that before she ventured out she had to be able to do everything on her own. She didn't want to deal with men coming up to her with a *Hey, little darling, looks like you need a strong man* attitude. This was why she'd learned to fix her own motorcycle when she'd traveled solo in her youth (she still rides it today but no longer takes it camping)—it kept her safer, and it avoided all that hassle. With this in mind, she watched YouTube videos and perused chat forums, and when she knew which nozzle went to what, the when and how of chocking wheels, the wherefore of dumping sewage, the whole RV shebang, only then did she load up and head out. "There was an oasis in Palm Springs I had heard about, and I wanted to hike it," she explains. After that she drove to Arizona. She avoided actual RV parks—she didn't like the way they teemed with people and exhaust fumes and noise. She parked near trailheads in small campgrounds and hiked all day. She wandered through art galleries in town, then back out to a trail. Did she miss Louie? I ask her. Of course she did, she answers. But she was also rejuvenated. And, surprisingly, joyful.

It seems counterintuitive to experience both grief and happiness simultaneously. But Pauline Boss knows that the very porousness of a certain kind of loss—"ambiguous loss," as she calls it—means that it necessarily makes room for other emotions, too. As Boss examines people grappling with a variety of absences, dissipations, and disappearances, she notes how loss can elude easy quantification. If your military spouse is declared missing in action, do you mourn a death or simply grieve an absence? If a loved one has dementia, how does one reckon with the way an old self has died while the body remains? In Illona's case, the loss of Louie was unambiguous—he died there, in the bedroom, in their house. Yet it also lingers in amorphous ways. Gone is the opportunity to cook for a partner who has just gallantly dumped the RV sewage. Gone is the security of knowing someone nearby will handle the kayaks. Gone is the identity of being a loving spouse. These are losses that are harder to see, and therefore to mourn. But as Boss iterates again and again, just because a loss is difficult to point to and pin down with a word or two, it doesn't mean it doesn't exist.

Illona long ago learned that on the road it's impossible to paint with her preferred medium of acrylic, so she taught herself to draw on her computer tablet; when she landed back home she would paint what she had sketched on her screen. She returned from her inaugural solo RV journey with an abundance of tablet images, and she even made wind chimes out of collected cactus skeletons. But since Louie's death she hasn't been able to actually paint, she tells me. Part of the problem is that she doesn't like being in the house, perhaps because that's where he died. She explains this lack of painting as if it is mostly just a sidebar to her current experience, but I recognize it clearly as another ambiguous loss.

After Louie died, Illona decided that it would be good to be more social—she likes being with people, and the final year of caretaking had been so lonely—so she signed up for an all-women hike "meetup." When she arrived at the trailhead everyone seemed to know each other. They clustered into informal groups, chattering; Illona knew nobody and stood off to one side quietly. On the trail the groups stayed intact; Illona hiked the whole day by herself. When the hike ended she thought to herself, Wow, I could've just done that alone. But she persevered, went back for the next one, made efforts to say hi, and gradually began to make connections. "I tell people now, if you do it this way with meetups, don't give up. It's strange at first. But you will make friends." Now she hikes once a week with the women. Most of them are younger than she is, but she likes that. It's difficult to find outdoorsy women her age, she tells me. Growing up female in her era, it was all *don't do sports, don't go on adventures, just get married, have a bunch of kids*, so it's no surprise to her. This, too, is something she does well: adapts.

We've come to the end of the marina. Ahead is a long seawall that leads to the mouth of the ocean. We could go all the way, but there is a small sandy beach on which more seals lie about, and we are happy to sit and watch them. An actual argument seems to be going on; a large—male?—seal has galumphed toward another—male?—and is roaring into his face, then sparring with his head and neck. The second seal soon slinks himself back into the water. A happier scene is playing out nearby—two smaller seals seem to be frolicking as they twist and turn just at the surface, though it's hard to be sure. To be in nature like this is to surrender most understanding and just observe, and that can be a relief.

As we rock gently on the water, paddles keeping us balanced, senses open, it occurs to me that we are mirroring Pauline Boss's outlook when she tells us that whatever loss we may be facing (a person, perhaps, or something more psychological, like the effects of a pandemic, or aging), it is not to be resolved; instead one must search for ways to live with it. It is a winding journey to *bear* loss rather than overcome it, and for this Boss offers advice:

> Look for meaning in the loss;
> Cede any notions of controlling what is uncontrollable;
> Adjust and solidify one's own identity;
> Make peace with ambiguity;
> Redefine the relationship with what or who one has been lost;
> Muster hope.

There are more honks and barks, and Illona and I float, watch, and listen. I'm elated when a flock of pigeons from a nearby dock scoots as a team over our heads so closely I can feel wingbeats. I appreciate that Illona is as happy to drift as she was to paddle the hour and a half to get here. I ask her how her relationship to the outdoors has changed with age. "I'm not in a rush to get anywhere," she muses. "I'm no longer as competitive. For me being outdoors is a way to be grateful for life. Everything is *beautiful.*"

We begin to head back, everything unfamiliar to me at this new angle. The ground fog has long burned off and the gray sky is now blue, adding to my bewilderment about the route. Illona keeps pointing to the direction of the ocean when I ask, but the winding waterways confound that terrible sense of direction I still have, so I finally just let her lead me home.

I came today to see how grief can be assuaged by getting outside. While nature is certainly a balm, I find that for Illona, it was all the necessary steps she took to access nature that also offered healing. The landscape became not just sea and trail, but a gentle proving ground that reconnected her to her confidence and sense of self, as she tackled the kayak rack, the RV, even the simple matter of leading a slightly disoriented companion along the marina. No big plans immediately, Illona tells me now as we paddle. Her life unfolds weekly instead, with certain days spent on the water, others in her garden, still others on a hiking trail. It is too soon to have a wider perspective on her Future, with a capital F. In due time, she will paint again. She will drive the RV to a new trailhead. Perhaps she will try a high mountain road, a few passes. Or perhaps not. We pull up to her tiny slip and before I know it she has hauled her kayak onto the dock and is fiddling with the locks on the rack as if she'd been doing this for years and years by herself, and not a YouTube video is in sight.

Join In

*Let me tell you what I think of bicycling. I think it has done more
to emancipate women than anything else in the world.*

—SUSAN B. ANTHONY, SUFFRAGETTE, SOCIAL REFORMER

Kittie Weston-Knauer puts on her helmet and instructs
me to do the same. Her helmet is the cool kind, with a
jutting protector around the lower half of her face, while mine
is a plain old bicycle helmet. In addition, Weston-Knauer, also
known as Miss Kittie, is wearing black canvas pants that hint
at wild crashes on asphalt, while I could only find a pair of
my mother's discarded Lycra bike leggings, complete with
crotch padding. All this makes clear that I don't know what
the heck I'm doing. Luckily, I am about to be taught by Miss
Kittie, who has been riding BMX bikes for thirty-five years.

In fact, at seventy-four years old, Miss Kittie is the oldest female BMX racer competing in the United States today.

I am here on this beautiful spring day, a little nervous, a little exhilarated, because I want to understand how a rigorous outdoor contest like BMX racing can benefit older women. Studies show that competitive sports help youth not just with physical fitness, but with social skills, leadership skills, self-confidence, and time management. This leads to more success in the classroom, and later, healthy boundaries. So why can't competitive sports help us as we age? BMX bike racing has a formality and a structure akin to say, triathlons, or the 5K running race for a cause that people gather and train for weekly, and I thought I could explore those similar outdoor activities through the lens of this lesser-known sport. To that end, Miss Kittie's plan today is not just to teach me to ride a BMX bike, but also to enroll me in the competition later that evening, so I can display my newfound skills to the families who gather weekly to engage in what she assures me is a low-key and friendly event.

Miss Kittie, who stands five feet, five inches tall, with a gap-toothed smile, tells me that she has also enlisted twelve-year-old Lucy Cooke for today's lesson, who will be arriving soon. Lucy is pitching in because, as Miss Kittie tells me, "Honey, kids are the best teachers." They don't fuss with big words or complicated concepts, she says, they just tell it like it is. This seems like Miss Kittie's style, too, which explains why she was in education her whole working life, retiring as a highly respected principal here in Des Moines, Iowa. Even now her talents as an educator are clear, as she eschews swear words while still getting her point across—she has already exclaimed "Son of a biscuit eater!" a few times and once sighed that she doesn't "give a fat rat." She also manages to turn things into teachable moments, as when she shrugs aside my admiration for her continual mentorship of girls in BMX with, "There's no sage on the stage, just a guide on the side, as I tell my kids." By "my kids" she means both her real, biological kids and her students.

Miss Kittie also wants twelve-year-old Lucy here because this is what BMX is all about. It's an intergenerational thing, with three-year-olds mounting pedal-less "strider bikes," their older siblings on cruisers and twenty-inchers, and their parents joining in. Well, the dads joining in, Miss Kittie tells me with a shake of her head. The moms rarely race. "Women tell me, 'I have so much going on,' and then I see their husband on the track and I say, 'Get your booty on the bike. Why should men have all the fun?'" This is the bane of Miss Kittie's existence, the lack of women in the sport. They may race as kids, but as soon as they finish high school, they tend to quit. Lucy holds the promise of how it could change for the future. This future, in Miss Kittie's eyes, must also include more people of color; as a Black woman, she is often the only nonwhite person on a bike at the race, she notes, and almost always the only female of color.

. . .

A BMX racetrack is a curlicue of dirt hummocks and asphalt berms. With as many as eight riders racing at a time, the goal is to simply burst out of the starting gate, negotiate the three turns, the various jumps and rollers in between, and the other bikes, and cross the finish line first. But along the way, a biker has to know when to pedal and when to simply pump the handlebars to get momentum, and how to take each turn.

This is why Miss Kittie and I walk the track as we wait for Lucy's arrival, Miss Kittie explaining the techniques as we go. Out of the gate, stay in your lane for at least thirty feet. Never sit down on the seat, that'll just get you in trouble (which is why Miss Kittie's pants have no crotch padding and I am walking around looking silly in these road-bike leggings). The hilly portion (also known as jumps and rollers, or "the rhythm section") needs some quick pedaling, then a succession of pulling up and pressing down on the handlebars to negotiate the lips. Coming into the first turn, "you want your line to be low to high or high to low," Miss Kittie says (by "line" she means the planned trajectory of your bike around the sloped corner). Hard pedal here. Don't pedal there (in certain places, pedals can catch on the ground, leading to a tumble). I ask what would happen if my high-low met someone else's low-high and she pauses to raise one eyebrow in the semiotics of school principals everywhere, wordlessly saying, Now do not disappoint me and crash, honey, okay?

Miss Kittie has been on a bike most of her life. She grew up in North Carolina, the third sibling of five brothers and a sister. "In our family, when you turned ten, you got your first bicycle. Well, you got your only bike, to be honest about it." It was the job of the older sibling to teach the next younger one, but when it was Kittie's time and her dad told her older brother to step up, "Martin said, 'Dad, Kittie has been riding my bike all along.'" She had taught herself, and why not? Bikes represented freedom, the ability to go anywhere. Biking "opened up the world," she says, "And the world was Durham, North Carolina." But it was, as Miss Kittie notes, a "tumultuous time," with civil rights in the South still a distant-seeming dream. She escaped by attending Drake University and then settled in Des Moines. She became a teacher and married, and she and her husband continued cycling family-style with their two sons. But it wasn't until one son, Max, was invited by a friend to a track that BMX came into their lives.

Miss Kittie, who also coached basketball and softball, was prone to yelling instructions at Max during his races. "I was on the sidelines saying You-ought-to-be, how-come-you're-not. And finally he said to his dad and me, 'If you think this is so easy why don't you try it?'" She put her money where her mouth was, or, as she might say, "I put Pat and Charley in the street" (meaning, her feet). On Mother's Day 1988, she got on Max's BMX bike. "I was hooked," she says. She was almost forty years old.

When I ask her why she found BMX so compelling, then and now, she says, "You need to learn something new every day on this earth, and I am still learning in the sport of BMX." Recently she was on a track that had dirt turns instead of the usual asphalt. She wasn't used to that, she tells me, and had to reassess the way she rode. "What did I have to do to be safe when I hit those turns?"

The physical fitness that comes with intense exertion is also important to her, she says. BMX cycling improves the heart and vascular system, with its fast bursts out of the gate and its steep hill climbs. It may even be considered weight-bearing, since there is no seat-sitting as in traditional riding, and thus it also helps the bones. And there is the camaraderie, she tells me. The race circuit takes her all over the country, where there "are so many interesting people to meet. Being able to have conversations with girls and women especially—you need to find something that allows you to continue to grow into old age. I won't race forever, but I'll be at the track forever." There is also the sense of adventure. "Hitting a turn at twenty miles per hour. Can you imagine that? That's where the exhilaration comes." Finally, she says, BMX biking is just plain fun. "If you aren't having fun every day, you're wasting your life."

As we walk and talk, Miss Kittie bends down to pick at the errant grasses that poke through the dirt. This is a community track, and it takes everyone pitching in to keep it running. She tells me she used to spend a full day at the school and then come here to weed. Though she has ridden some tracks as short as 700 feet and others as long as 1,300 feet, this track is average length; that's 995 feet of weeding, Miss Kittie says. When I ask how long it takes to ride—two minutes, five minutes?—she laughs. "I hope not! That's long enough for a nap." It'll be under a minute, she assures me. "So, no getting air and jumping and twisting?" I persist, which turns out to be a different use of the BMX bike. Miss Kittie pulls a weed and tells me I've been watching way too much TV.

Lucy bounds up, all smiles and energy, tall for her age, Caucasian, with freckles, bright blue eyes, and long brown hair. She and Miss Kittie banter about the past weekend, where they participated in separate races, Miss Kittie in Cedar Rapids, Lucy and her family in Fort Wayne, Indiana—her older brother and four younger siblings (the youngest still on a strider bike) race as well. Lucy tells us she won her first heat (called a "moto" in BMX lingo), which consisted of all boys because there weren't any other girls to race against. In the second moto, she crashed and hurt her ribs. She didn't want to stop racing, though, so her father simply wrapped her rib cage. The next day she was back on the bike and came in second. Her ribs were almost broken, she was told later.

"You continued to race?" I say, incredulous.

Both Lucy and Miss Kittie look at me as if I had jabbed one of their bike tires with a pen.

"Yes," Lucy says, shrugging.

"You don't just stop because of a sore this or that," agrees Miss Kittie. "Could you imagine? I would not be racing, period." There are actually many reasons Miss Kittie should, in theory, not be racing, period. She has suffered from osteoarthritis since she was in her twenties, which makes her joints hurt and which may explain why she walks with a forward tilt and a piratelike gait, legs sweeping outward as if to accommodate a scabbard at her side. Then, about ten years ago, she began the process of replacing both hips and both knees. She told the doctor each time that she needed to be healed by racing season, so she had the operations in successive winters and was ready to get back on the bike each April. But surgeries are nothing compared to the accident she had just a few years into racing, at age forty-five. Attempting to learn how to jump, her pedal caught and she pitched forward. She broke her neck, "a C-4-5 break, like Christopher Reeve. And he was Superman, and totally paralyzed. The doctor told my husband, 'I don't think she'll have full use of her limbs.' And I said, 'I'm going to walk on out of this hospital.'" And she did.

Miss Kittie talks about the ensuing couple of years as if they were a gift, not an excruciating procession of slow nerve regeneration in her feet and long hours of physical therapy ("You could bounce a quarter off my thighs, I was so ripped," she says). She was determined to "use this accident, this experience, as a lesson to help students understand that there was nothing in the world you couldn't do if you put your mind to it."

As she recovered, she began to lurk around the track. "I was walking around with a collar on my neck, wanting to qualify for Worlds." In September 1994, a year after the accident, there she was at the starting line for the World Championship 41–45 Men's Cruiser class; she had to race against men because there were no women from any countries in that age group. Of her fellow racers, she says, "They were shocked that a woman was there. That a woman of *color* was there." She didn't advance after the first round of motos, but she did beat a British man who later came up to tell her how impressed he was. (In the 2007 Worlds, racing against women in the 45 and Over Cruiser class, fifty-nine-year-old Miss Kittie finished in seventh place.)

Miss Kittie has been asked many times why she continued after such a close call with paralysis. "My answer to them is, 'Why not?' As long as I can keep the two wheels on the ground, I'm going to keep doing it." She loved BMX racing, so instead of quitting, she simply changed the way she raced. She doesn't tangle with anyone on the corners or go handlebar to handlebar on the straights. She'll pull back in order not to engage. Her objective these days is to compete, do her best, and not crash. Adaptation, she tells me, is always the key. She shows me her latest bike ("my last bike"), which she paid no small sum for, she tells me, constructed to accommodate the knees, the hips, and everything else as she ages. It's light, with shocks to absorb the bumps. The tires are wide. It has pink cables. There are components like the Spank Tweet Tweet bar, the Alienation billy club, Ruffian grips. No doubt this is a bike that prompts a low whistle from any serious BMX rider; it bristles with capability.

. . .

We pull out the bike I will be riding from the back of her van. It belonged to her husband, Max, who died in 2019, a pretty blue-and-white deal that looks almost new. I ask if she's sure it's okay; I'm a beginner, after all, and it seems like a special bike. She waves me off. "Well, it is. But you know, it's just a bike, baby."

Lucy doesn't seem fazed by the idea of spending the afternoon teaching an older adult how to ride the track; she actually seems psyched. Miss Kittie instructs us first to take a spin in the parking lot to see if I can really ride. ("You'd be surprised how many people can't," she tells me.) Once I pass that test, Lucy says she'll follow me around the track. She dons her helmet (with its chin protector and Darth Vader menace) and we push our bikes up a tall manmade hill to the starting line. Perched there, I warily eye the steep grade before me while Lucy explains the gates (though we won't be using them at first): the rider's front tire presses forward against the steel, a countdown begins, she balances up on her pedals, the gates drop, she pedals like a maniac.

Many riders have a nickname that they emblazon on their racing jersey. You have to earn it though, Lucy "Tough Cookie" Cooke tells me. (Some other examples of nicknames include Charlie "Choo-choo" Townsend; Dino "Bazooka" Deluca, and the stand-alone and much-used "Psycho.") I haven't earned a nickname yet, but silently I wonder if a placeholder nickname is allowed. Something humble, something descriptive.

Tough Cookie turns to Caroline "The Writer" Paul.

"Ready?" she asks me.

"Yes," I say.

"Let's go," she answers.

I stomp down, trying to do my puny version of a fast start. Lucy drops in behind. "Pedal hard!" she shouts. My legs— knees stiff and often inflamed from past surgeries, ankle permanently tweaked—are not the strongest part of me; my version of pedaling hard feels like slow motion. But it's enough to propel me down the steep starting hill, then up, hitting the tabletop at a speed that makes it seem as if I'm getting air. I let out what can only be a little squeal (a video I watch later confirms that no, there was no air. There was a squeal.) "Pedal, pedal, into the first turn," Lucy is now saying, whereupon I pedal twice, then brake hard, making another strange sound with my throat.

"You're doing good!" she encourages me into the new set of rollers. "Pump!"

"Pump!" I respond, bringing the bike through into the next turn, making loud exhale noises for no reason I can discern. Lucy keeps up the encouraging banter as the final turn looms, the tightest of them all. But there is nothing like a twelve-year-old saying "Nice!" and "Good job!" as if she means it to give you undeserved confidence. The curve is survived without a mishap. I bounce through the final rollers. One more "Pedal, pedal!" from Lucy and we are over the finish line. This was so much more fun than I expected, and as I slow I whoop. We dismount. Lucy gives me a high five.

"You did good!" she says (this, even though the video shows that I resemble Gumby on a bike). We push our bikes back to the start.

After a few runs Miss Kittie joins us on the track and now the three of us pedal around. I'm not supposed to go all out, but in my excitement I forget, not to mention that my "all out" is their version of a practice run. After a couple of laps, my legs begin to feel a little wobbly. I wonder how it would be to have eight riders at once jostling for position. Miss Kittie says that there have been some "hellified races" with the men-over-forty age group, but she stays clear of all that. And there are rarely many women in a local race anyway. In an odd twist, I will actually be racing both Lucy and Miss Kittie in what is supposed to be the 46–50 Women's Cruiser class, but has now reverted to just the Women's Cruiser class, because out of the fifty or so racers tonight the three of us are the only females on cruiser bikes (bikes in this race have twenty-four inch wheels. Otherwise, there are a few young girls racing in the class races, which use the standard twenty-inch-wheeled bike. Lucy is also racing in those).

"Women will especially tell you 'I can't,'" Miss Kittie explains with a frown. We are sitting by her van in foldout red chairs, our helmets nearby, the bikes against a tree. "But there is only 'I don't want to' or 'Try to make me.'" She doesn't buy the excuses, and there are many. Some women say they can't afford it. "I say, 'Are you drinking or smoking cigarettes? I don't care, but for every pack of cigarettes, instead of paying that kind of money, put it in a jar, and [soon] you'll be able to afford it, honey.'" Others tell her there is simply no time. She understands: "Here's what we do as women: we take care of everyone except ourselves," she says. But ultimately, she doesn't buy this excuse, either. Working at the school until 7:00 P.M., she and her husband, Max, also an educator, still found time to race as a family. Her son JP, who is nonverbal autistic, she explains, never wanted to race, but on weekends all four of them piled into the RV, ultimately traveling all over the United States and Canada. Those long car rides were an unexpected boon, allowing her to spend time with her kids. It made her a better mother, Miss Kittie tells me. "I had a young man [Max] who was growing up. No, no, no, I'm not going to be his friend. But you do things together. And I brought JP along and people got to know him."

The race area is beginning to fill up with families, who spill from their vans and trucks and SUVs. They set up shade structures and crack open sodas. They buy chips from the shipping container turned concession stand, and many of them come over to where Miss Kittie and I are sitting, to pay their respects. Miss Kittie, it turns out, is famous. Not just as a BMXer, but as a teacher and as a person. Some of the people who approach she's known since they were kids on the track. Others were in her classroom. At one point, a young woman introduces herself and mentions that Miss Kittie taught her brother, who is doing well in Tennessee right now, after a rough start as a kid. Miss Kittie remembers. After all, she was the kind of teacher—the last of this kind of teacher, probably—who did home visits. Her final job was as principal in an alternative school where "I got the gangbangers, I got the kids coming out of prison. Kids who'd been in fights wound up with me. And there were kids catching up on their credits." Now Miss Kittie listens closely, then says, "I heard he was doing well, I'm so glad, honey. And what about you, baby, what are you doing?"

At another point, a ten-year-old appears with a shy smile. "Are you Miss Kittie?" he asks. He introduces himself and then tells her that he and his family came today just to see her ride. She leaves me to go shake hands with the mom and dad and siblings. She is determined to get them on the track, especially the mom, who rides bikes seriously anyway. This happens every race, the influx of fans, especially when she is on the road. "It's good for BMX," she says, shrugging. "But don't idolize me. I put on my pants one leg at a time, same as you."

Miss Kittie travels to events all over the Midwest and the East. Most years she competes in around fifty to sixty races; many are local, like today's, but some have impressive names like the Gold Cup, the Triple Point, and Race of Champions. She loads up and drives a twenty-nine-foot RV (that's even longer than Illona's RV, and the height of a gabled two-story building). Once at the racetrack she camps—and she does this on her own: Max, her husband, is gone, of course. Max, her son (Max IV, technically), lives out of state, no longer races, and is married with three children, while JP lives in a home for intellectually challenged adults, she explains. Miss Kittie isn't intimidated by traveling alone, though if the races are in the South, she is more careful. "You wouldn't believe what still goes on, honey," she says. She shakes her head at the thought of being a Black person all alone on those country roads. "When I do go, I only go to races just off an exit, right off the highway."

Despite the persistent bigotry in this country, Miss Kittie believes in the power of BMX racing to provide health, a sense of purpose, and fellowship. But mostly she believes simply in the power of the bike. With the blessing of the Des

Moines city council, Miss Kittie teams up every year with officers from the Police Activity League and together they host a bike camp for local kids, ages eleven to fifteen. The kids bring their own bikes and basic riding skills (along with "good physical health and positive behavior" and "athletic attire—no sandals," as the flyer reads). They learn bike maintenance, bike safety, the proper use of gears. It's not BMXing, but it's an important class, Miss Kittie says, because a bike teaches kids responsibility, and it gives them independence and freedom. She hopes they will bike to school, bike with friends. She hopes they will wheel around the perimeter of their own world with confidence, getting there safely and with the ability to fix what gets broken, then peer beyond that world with resolve and wonder, as she once did.

The track announcer—a volunteer, like everyone else here—shouts through a megaphone that the races will begin soon, so we don our helmets and gloves and cinch tight our leggings. We wheel our bikes to the gate. I don't like competition, to be honest. But everything about today seems to be about fun, not winning, starting with the fact that I am lining up against the two people who just generously taught me how to ride the course in the first place.

We are side by side in our lanes. Miss Kittie has gone quiet, concentrating. The gate is upright. Lights flash, the announcer says something about Miss Kittie, Lucy Cooke, and Caroline Paul, an author all the way from California, then the gate drops. I'm slow off the start. Both Lucy and Miss Kittie are ahead. I catch Miss Kittie at a roller, but Lucy is far gone. I'm still in second by the next turn. Push? Pull? I confuse the order of my pumping and seem to come to a stop at the top of the next roller, then manage to creep over it. Pedaling hard now,

I zip toward the final turn. I'm grinning and talking to myself. Pedal! Brake! Pump! It's all over in fifty-three seconds.

In all, we race three motos and each one is pretty much the same. I'm the last out of the gate. Miss Kittie lets me pass her before the first turn. (I know this because on the second moto, we reach that first turn at the same time and she says, "Go on, now, baby, you take it.") It's not that she is trying to be nice. No, Miss Kittie is competitive, and she's always charging to do her best. It's more that it isn't worth it for her to mix it up with a rank beginner on a corner—no crashing for Miss Kittie. So each time I blunder ahead and keep the lead. Twelve-year-old Tough Cookie is a blur ahead of both of us. No one in the crowd really pays attention. Miss Kittie and I approach a sizzling (in my book) 17.4 mph, according to Miss Kittie's speedometer. Ultimately, I earn a second-place trophy, if not a real nickname yet.

When I first interviewed Miss Kittie, I was sure that my quest was to go deep on how competition invigorates us as we age. The BMX world had seemed a colorful template, especially gritty and macho, with an audience bloodthirsty for brawling wheels on the straightaways, shoulder bumps in turns, and spectacular crackups. Whoever came out on top would be revered, certainly. How would that sharpen our gaze, fire up our neurons, I wondered? But nowhere is any of that on display today. The watchword on the BMX track is more "fun" than "win." Miss Kittie herself let me pass her on the turn. She is competitive, sure, but not if it means getting hurt. That's not to say that the BMX community doesn't appreciate a good race. There are many aspects of competition at play. There is the camaraderie, the goal setting (Lucy has her eye on the Olympics), the physical challenge, the way you can gather with your friends and just whiz around. In fact, to become a BMX bike racer is similar to becoming a runner or a triathlete, especially when you decide to engage in these competitive sports through a large local group or regular meetup.

"Happy people tend to spend more time with others," says Yale University cognitive scientist Laurie Santos, also known as the Happiness Professor. "This is one of the clearest things we see from the science." It is not just the human connection that provides the well-being, though, but what studies call "the sense of community belonging" or simply "belonging needs." This deeper feeling of cohesion is why outdoor activities like BMX can be so sustaining, also offering us what Santos calls a "cultural apparatus" to get outside ourselves and our own problems. She says that much modern self-care, with its inward focus and advice to concentrate on massage routines and personal downtime, may actually be self-defeating; a better happiness regimen is to, say, line up on a starting line with a group of like-minded speed enthusiasts, or take a new BMX biker under your wing.

It's worth reiterating here that so many of the women I've talked with only later realize how much the community aspect of their outdoor adventure adds to its impact. When I interviewed triathlete Joan Wicks, fifty-nine, she told me she had at first specifically rejected anything that involved other people. It was 2018, and she knew she "needed something to jump-start my life physically." She was fifty-five years old and suddenly an empty nester—her twin daughters, one of whom is presidential inauguration poet Amanda Gorman, the other filmmaker Gabrielle Gorman—had left the house for college. Why did she still have so little energy? She needed to be more active, she decided, but didn't want to rely on anybody else to complete her goals. Running, she decided, might be the antidote, requiring only a pair of sneakers and a safe place outside to train. And also, in her case, an app called Couch to 5K, which organized her workouts for her and promised to get her running 5K in three months. It actually took her five months—five torturous, never-ending, but somehow satisfying months, at the end of which she considered herself if not a runner, at least someone who could run. She jogged on her own for a while, then signed up with a running group called the LA Leggers that met every Saturday to race. It was their race expertise that she was interested in; the community aspect wasn't on her radar, she tells me. But at her very first Leggers' Saturday, her pace group—all strangers—waited for her at the finish line, cheering her on and taking pictures. Something sparked.

When I asked Joan how being part of a community changed her, she replied, "I started becoming one of those people that shows up. I'm not saying that I wasn't that person before, but when it comes to exercise—'It's cold outside'; 'Oh, I don't feel like getting out of bed'—no, you become the person that gets out of bed at 4:45 A.M. even if it's raining. So, you develop a different level of, I guess, perseverance, resilience, determination, and it just becomes part of you."

I was especially intrigued that Joan didn't stop pushing, not even when she joined the 5:30 A.M. workouts with the group Black Girls Run, often running five miles before a full workday, nor after her first marathon (where somehow she missed all the aid stations and, famished, asked a woman on the sidelines for her croissant). Instead, she kept looking wider and farther for a challenge, and hit upon triathlons. By that point, Joan fully understood the power of training with other people. Which was good, because her new sport required that she become proficient in not just one sport but the triad of swimming, running, and biking, not to mention the tricks of the trade that help a racer transition between the three. Of her new life exercising with others outside, she tells me, "I call it grown-up day camp. . . . It's a second childhood, that's what it feels like. And we're having a blast."

BMX and triathlons have much in common. They are both competitive arenas, with medals and personal bests of which to boast. Also, while neither are team sports per se, the experience is still communal. What sets BMX apart, however, is how the ages mix and mingle. Just last weekend it was Lucy's sister, five-year-old Hazel, chatting with Miss Kittie in one of the red camp chairs instead of me (the proof is in the blurry chocolate-chip-cookie-and-apple-juice-ish stain on the seat). This seems totally normal to both Hazel and Miss Kittie, but I can't think of another sport where that happens so easily. Nor another sport where I would be mentored enthusiastically by both a twelve-year-old and a seventy-four-year-old.

One of my favorite Miss Kittie-isms is "Every time I get on my bike I win." Like all her sayings, this is not flip. After all, Miss Kittie is not supposed to be here at the BMX track, in so many ways. As a woman, as an elder woman, as a woman of color, as a survivor of a traumatic accident. And yet, here she is. She knows she's the keeper of a flame, and a role model, an educator in a new kind of school. People look up to her, women especially. Kids look up to her. In this way, she is following her family tradition when it comes to bikes, and metaphorically teaching the next youngest how to ride.

Ultimately, Miss Kittie has had to learn to transcend winning itself, because there is no one her age to race against anymore. Years before, she had petitioned the two national BMX associations to add adult women cruiser races, and was successful, but the women still hang back. Miss Kittie doesn't give up hope, but for now it's her versus . . . nobody, really. She pedals only against doubts that she should be on the track to begin with. That seems the most important competition of all.

Miss Kittie is determined to age gracefully. "Gracefully means I am still active and engaged and involved. I don't know what my body is going to be, but I'm not going to complain, 'Oh, Miss Kittie, it's awful . . . I can't do this, I can't do that.' I will always have a good time." She understands that there may be a day when she will no longer ride. But until that day, she will race against whoever shows up, pushing her bike to the starting line, hearing the names announced, lining up. The lights will flash, the riders will be ready. Into that suddenly quiet moment before the pandemonium of legs and tires will slide the creak of a bike being balanced, the slight sibilance of a brake pressed, and the whisper of humans breathing almost in unison, before the gate drops.

Be Ready for Change

I find the lure of the unknown irresistible.

—Sylvia "Her Deepness" Earle, age 86,
MARINE BIOLOGIST AND DIVE LEGEND

There's no way around it: the weather sucks. Wind from the wrong direction, whitecaps, gray skies. As an even bigger swell approaches, I brace myself with a forward paddle stroke. I'm on what is called a stand-up paddleboard (SUP), but I'm not standing—I've been paddling on my knees for the past twenty minutes, hoping the angle or height of the waves will somehow change. But no, here they are slapping at me from the side, getting as high as three feet. I'm not new to SUPs, but I am new to paddling so long like this. Once or twice I gamely clamber to my feet, take a few strokes, see a

large wave heading my way, and sink back down, clutching
at the heavy gear bag strapped to the bow and filled with items
necessary for a night of camping. The wave hits. The board
dips and slides, and my arms shoot skyward for balance. Then
it has passed, with another heading my way. Weather changes,
the sages say. This is supposed to be a deeply comforting
maxim. But right now, the weather is changing for the worse,
with the wind rising and the sky a roiling gray.

Sometimes I love the outdoors for its rigorous demands.
But sometimes I just plain wish it would be sunny and calm.
I am holding both thoughts right now. The concentration
it is taking to stay upright allows me to be intensely in the
moment, which is rare while onshore going about my day.
But I'm also getting tired, these bumbling dance moves
I'm doing taking their toll. Luckily, I'm enduring this with
few spectators on this section of Lake Tahoe, as it's late in the
day and the weather so uninviting; there are just some faraway
motorboaters who throw up wake without looking my way,
and, on another paddleboard ahead of me, my good friend Sue
Norman.

Sue is sixty-five, but you can't tell when you look at her;
her skin has none of the wrinkles you would expect from a
white girl who has been outdoors so much. Her dangling
earrings give her a slight hippie vibe, but that's confounded
by the Patagonia jacket and surf shorts. She has no gray in her
short light-brown hair that I can see, and she doesn't dye it,
either, and because she just can't be bothered otherwise, she
used to trim it with a pair of dog clippers (she assures me that
these days she gets a haircut in town). Finally, to cap off her
agelessness, she is still impossibly lean from years of backcountry skiing, as well as SUP racing on this very lake. I add

this last point because it's worth noting that she, too, is now paddling from a kneeling position; if these conditions are kicking her butt a little, I don't feel so bad. It's not the height of the waves, really, but the fact that they are hitting us from the side that is the problem. "We never get an east wind in summer!" Sue shouts over to me, shaking her head. "I didn't expect this!"

The fact that today's weather catches Sue by surprise reminds me how much things have changed. Sue was once someone who always had a plan, and she executed that plan with precision and success. Her friends affectionately called her Sarge for this keen eye on logistics, and her insistence that details and a schedule be followed to a T. *Hey Sarge, what's the plan? Whatever you say, Sarge, on the double.* Now I wonder what else is up for grabs on our camping trip today, what else could catch us unaware, that we've overlooked. (Rain, it turns out. Also, possibly, bears.)

Behind Sue is her little dog Pearl, resplendent in a red and yellow life jacket, looking unhappy. Her rat terrier legs are wide; she has gotten the hang of balancing, but it's clear she doesn't understand why her human wants to be out here. Every so often water sprays up from the sides, and Pearl half closes her eyes and turns her head with the repressed outrage of a nun. Behind both of us is a twelve-year-old: Seth, who is also my godson, has the luxury of being in a much more stable and much faster boat—called a one-person ocean canoe, or an OC-1 for short. Sue yells above the wind for him to hurry up; in response, he languidly dips his paddle into the water, and then sits back and looks around. He's not worried about tipping or falling off—the hull is narrow but braced by a long outer arm called the amah, allowing it to remain mostly impervious to the cumbersome conditions—and he's making it clear in that preteen way that paddling near us is a bore.

I decide to again try to stand. I clamber up successfully, take a few strokes. But the wave trains keep advancing. Within only a few moments the SUP begins to wobble, and I do a few inelegant stutter steps. There is a moment of suspension, and I teeter between balance and imbalance. Then I'm in the water. The board is unfazed, floating upright, the camp gear safe in its special dry bag; it's just me who is wet. The beauty of the SUP is this very gentility—easy to load onto a car, easy to paddle, easy to scramble aboard again.

Kneeling remains the best option, I decide.

Sue learned to fend for herself early; her mother had developed a debilitating form of multiple sclerosis when she and her twin brother were still very young. Their overwhelmed father did his very best, but two kids and a sick wife was too much, and by the time the twins were ten years old it was agreed that their mom would be cared for elsewhere. Money was tight, but on weekends Sue's dad would bundle the twins up, throw a canoe on the roof of the station wagon, and drive to a river. He was a Lewis and Clark history buff, so these excursions often followed their trail, even when it meant accidentally paddling down dangerous sections of white water. There was one especially harrowing wipeout, when Sue and her brother, David, clung to the top of the overturned canoe and their father straddled the nose, cursing God and steering as best he could through three miles of gnarly white water. Despite this, or maybe because of it, Sue learned early to love outdoor adventure.

If you want structure in your life, you either throw yourself into a serious sport or you enlist in the military. Sue did both. She and David joined the army after high school. David didn't like it and was eventually discharged, but Sue took to the rigor and routine. She held many jobs while there, including clerk, military police officer, and also trainer of military police dogs. Despite her nickname of Sarge, she wasn't actually a sergeant, rising instead to the equivalent of corporal (technically it was Specialist Fourth Class). While stationed in Germany, she parlayed childhood river experiences into teaching other army personnel how to kayak. Soon she was a competitive kayaker in both the white water slalom and wildwater events, eventually becoming one of the top five in the United States, competing all over the world on the national team. In these early years she had boyfriends who swooned over her girl-next-door good looks, but by the time I met her, when she was in her late twenties, she'd realized she was a lesbian. She planned her life from there—a college degree, a good job, ownership of a small house, a few dogs, serious girlfriends who were themselves independent and outdoorsy, a future pension, and lots of time off to enjoy her skiing, paddling, surfing, and hiking adventures. Marriage and kids were unusual for gay people at the time, and that was fine for her—certainly it made mapping out the future so much easier. As a planner myself, I've always admired Sue's planning skills, but I gathered early that her interest in a known path forward came from a deep place—a need for the financial and emotional security she hadn't had as a child. So "Sarge" was born, and proceeded to lead a life of enviable adventure, with a clear, unwavering vision for the future.

I've known Sue for almost forty years—we met through river friends from my days as a whitewater guide for a dinky weekend rafting company. We bonded over a shared love of animals and reading, her boundless curiosity and deep intelligence, a need for more female friends who loved the outdoors, and, eventually, mutually flexible work schedules that allowed for overseas wilderness expeditions (I became a firefighter and she a hydrologist for the Forest Service). Even though we have always lived in separate places, we see each other when we can, so it's not unusual to find us on a lake together. But I am here today for a specific reason: as Sue neared sixty, her once finely tuned trajectory changed drastically. Aging often throws wrenches at the life plan, and Sue's plan was especially tight, the change especially abrupt. I'm here to see if she can help me understand how the outdoors played a part in adjusting, learning, and eventually embracing that.

Sue now lifts her paddle and assures me that the camp spot is just past *that point*. I can see the rock outcropping, and it doesn't look far, but I stay on my knees. Then she turns back to Seth and shouts over the wind, "You would never guess that you are in one of the fastest human-powered boats in the world." He pretends not to hear her. I tease, pointing out he is still only twelve, so why is he acting like a teenager? "I was so sweet when I was your age," I say, fibbing only a little. "It wasn't until I was thirteen that I stopped talking to pretty much anyone." Just as I hoped, I am rewarded with a boy's half smile. But he's still annoyed, and calls out to Sue, his voice breaking with puberty, but resonant with the whine of young kids everywhere:

"Mom, when are we going to get there?"

Mom?

In her fifties, Sue's life suddenly quit unspooling as planned. Call it what you will, an errant east wind perhaps; her twin brother, David, became an unexpected father at age fifty-two. His partner was twenty years old, with two other children, already overwhelmed. The two struggled with separate personal crises, and the household, Sue could tell, was deteriorating. She began to read about child development, and realized that at three years of age there was little time left wherein Seth could emerge from the difficulties of his upbringing relatively unscathed, and she stepped in. By stepped in, I really mean *leaped*. She asked for legal guardianship. Both David and Seth's mother saw what Sue could offer: stability, discipline, security. Sue filed the paperwork. She was Aunt Sue to Seth at first, but soon she became Mom.

It's hard to overstate just how big a swerve this was. Yes, there are many older people in this country who have to take on the responsibility of, say, their grandchildren. They think that their days of raising kids are over, but then their own children can't cope, getting involved in drugs, landing in jail, or battling mental health issues. The difference here is that Sue had never been a mother. She had no kids in her life at all. Her friends were almost exclusively child-free. They were outdoorsy types, routinely heading off for difficult backcountry ski lines or international wilderness expeditions. Similarly, Sue worked set hours, embarked on outdoor adventures, then schemed her next outdoor adventure. She and her wife, Lisa, a photographer, even lived apart about half the time, in the houses they owned before their marriage. This way each could immerse themselves in separate passions—Lisa rode horses at a nearby stable, and Sue could just about ski out her own back door into wilderness. In sum, Sue led the most chaos-free, highly predictable life one can imagine. The arrival of Seth, then, was much like that of Moses in a papyrus basket, stuck in the reeds of the Nile River, found by the pharaoh's daughter. You might as well have included booming decrees and flashes of lightning; Sue's transformation into a mother at fifty-six years old felt almost biblical.

Suddenly it was thrown toys, the right foods, strict eight o'clock bedtimes, a search for a preschool. Sue, so competent on a steep ski slope or a fast-moving river, found herself overwhelmed by this new landscape. She looked around for support and, frankly, couldn't find it. There may be some mythical world where a posse of parents bond and watch their children grow up together, but how could that happen here? She was thirty years older than the mothers and fathers around her. Parenting, Sue found out quickly, was not only stressful. It was exceedingly lonely.

Sue tells me now how much she misses her old friends, many of whom could not adjust to this new Sue. No longer free. No longer reliable (there is no other person who cancels plans more often than a parent, shackled as they are to sudden sinus infections, babysitter turmoil, and school outings). No longer Sarge. They dialed back interactions; many peeled away completely. Even the few friends who did have children—now so much older, of course—seemed to recoil, as if they didn't want to be dragged back from the place in their own (possibly difficult) parenting journey.

I don't escape this analysis, either: I wasn't the attentive friend I should have been. I didn't live nearby, yet why didn't I check in more often, make plans to visit with more frequency? I can only think that in my own (kidless) way, I too was totally thrown by this new Sue, gallant but discombobulated.

After all, didn't Sue's situation make it starkly clear how precarious a life plan could be, and didn't this just freak the fuck out of us? If this kind of disruption could happen to Sarge, surely the rest of us didn't stand a chance. Just as we are settling into our hard-won later life, certain of our trajectory, our shoulder is grabbed and we are spun around to face the simple fact that *shit happens*. The fates would have their way with us, too, her situation seemed to say, and this scared the bejesus out of us. What was around our next corner? A falling piano, a banana peel, a doctor's X-ray?

I'm presenting this new stage in Sue's life as if it was thrust upon her. This is simply the way I initially digested it. She *chose* to step in, of course. But how much of a choice is it if you've already made yourself into the person you want to be by your mid-fifties, and that person is loyal and brave? *Of course* Sue was going to intervene. It was murkier for her wife, Lisa, who was surely even more blindsided by this turn of events than Sue herself. She was serious and quiet, someone for whom the only reasonable chaos was that of her dogs running mad, merry circles in her living room, and not even that for long. Yes, she took breathtaking photos of wild mustangs for a living, and they often featured fighting stallions and herds at a gallop. But these frenetic, ferocious scenes were all stopped midstride and midkick, beautiful renderings of wildness that in no way resembled the feral antics of a real human child, say, before bedtime. Lisa agreed—tentatively at first—to stand by Sue. They would try it: raise Seth together. There were two houses, after all; that might take the edge off, they both hoped. Sue thought that Lisa would leave in those early years, she confesses to me. Instead Lisa became another adult role model and steady beacon of love and caring for Seth.

I jump off the board in the shallows, unload my gear bag. My knees have indents from the rubber padding I've been kneeling on. Pearl has been eyeing me bitterly this whole trip, but now she is running circles in the sand. Sue and Seth are tussling over the care and handling of the OC-1, which is a delicate boat. Sue is stern with him, and he claps back, as preteens do, but in the next second seems to have forgotten the admonishment. Seth doesn't hold grudges and has always been an essentially happy kid. As I watch the two together I notice how he has sprouted up recently, taller than Sue, gangly, with a floppy head of hair and a slouch. I ask him to sing a song from the theater camp he is attending, but he reddens and declines.

Sue may have always been a little tightly wound, but since being a parent that has surged into full-blown bouts of anxiety. She confides that she wakes up in the middle of most nights, suddenly fearful. She worries about Seth. She worries about the state of his world. She worries about his future jobs, his future friends, and the technologies that alienate. (I never thought the word "screen" would so permeate her vocabulary, as in "no more screens today.") And yet, while these past years have been full of anxiety, Sue says over and over that adopting Seth has also been the best and most important decision of her life. She wouldn't trade it for anything in the world. She is, in all these ways, a typical parent. Except that she is at a strange and unique crossroads where she is dealing both with the worries of a much younger person and also the anxieties of someone who is sixty-four.

"I've been thinking a lot about growing old. It's tough on all these levels I've never before understood," Sue tells me. She spends a lot of time battling feelings of irrelevance. Whether that is because she is aging in a country that doesn't value older women, or because she has lost her main social group, or because she is simply subsumed by raising a young boy, is hard to parse. Sue may look a good decade younger than she is, but she laments that she can no longer keep up with the forty-something kayakers, say, or crank out the ski climbs like she used to. Add to all that the difficulty of trying to hang out with young moms. "That's just awkward," she says, laughing ruefully. Her background in nature helps, she tells me, because the outdoors has always made her feel inconsequential, but in an uplifting, existential way. She says, "If you're outdoors a lot you become more comfortable with your place in the world, because, really, nature just doesn't care."

During Seth's younger years, Sue found that the wilderness made a good playground, and she and Seth would often embark on small excursions. In this way, while Seth burned off his incandescent energy, she could pivot into familiar terrain and shrug off some of the stresses of parenthood. They rode horses. They sledded. They swam. They rafted down rivers and paddled across lakes.

But neighborhood life had changed since Sue was a child—she was surprised to find that even in this mountain town kids didn't seem to spontaneously play in the streets or gather on someone's stoop in a pack to amuse themselves with stickballs or marbles or fort building. Instead, they were micromanaged into soccer games and baseball camps. Sue decided that if she couldn't find that imagined neighborhood, she would make it herself; these past few years she has taken to inviting kids Seth's age and their families to her beautiful but untamed, slightly mangy even, property an hour away, in the Sierra foothills. She might not even know the kids' families well but banks on the outdoors to facilitate bonding. The focal point on this piece of land is a big pond on which

I once watched the kids that she had gathered play a game that looked like "step on the back of the paddleboard until you fall off," with rules discernible only to those under ten, because every now and then someone would cry, "I won!" The kids later ran off to look at goats and play Uno in a horse corral. The parents sat in folding chairs under the fading light, paying no attention to their offspring, who floated by only as disembodied squeals and shouts now and then, and that was enough. Even Sue seemed to shed some of her anxiety. "I believe in the power of free play," she explained to me once, and there I saw it happening, in real time, for both adults and children alike.

I shrug off my wet life jacket and survey our temporary home. It's a sandy spit just inside a bay, surrounded by high mountain peaks. The beach is only fifteen yards wide or so, giving way to thick Sierra forest. A fishing boat idles just offshore, but otherwise we are alone. The wind has dropped. The clouds unfold and regroup, then unfold again as dusk approaches, and I hold on to the hope they will clear completely. When it gets dark I want to point out some constellations, really my only party trick of any note. As I am Seth's godmother, surely this is one of my responsibilities. He should be able to spot the Big Dipper. He should know the North Star. If we're lucky and the clouds relent, we can also gawk at my favorite star, Antares, flashing its magnificent beacon of green-yellow-red on the horizon.

Our dinner is simple: burritos and jelly beans. We haven't brought forks, or a stove, or a tent for that matter. Instead: a change of clothes, a flashlight, a sleeping bag and pad, a few protein bars. A rain poncho will double as a groundsheet. This is lean and mean camping, no fuss. I did secretly pack my pillow, and a camp chair, despite Sue instructing me not to, and I have a thermos of coffee for the morning. ("I have a new motto," I tell her in defense. "It's *Why be tortured.*) The plan is to stay the night, then wake up in the morning and explore this bay. Then we will depart to civilization in time to get Seth to his afternoon theater camp. This is a typical outdoor adventure for Sue these days. Minimal logistics, with leeway for Seth's commitments.

How things have changed. Well before the internet made it so much easier, I could rely on Sue to dream up an outlandish expedition and then scrupulously lay out the route and details. She has been a friend that way above all, inviting me on adventures I would not have planned on my own. We have sea kayaked for weeks among the islands of Belize. We've set up tents on wild beaches in Baja, surfing during the day. We snow-camped, skinning up empty wilderness slopes and skiing down. We once paddled stand-up boards along the lee side of Catalina Island for three days, camping along the way. We were new to paddleboards, and certainly to camping with them. We had to jury-rig the best way to carry our gear, resulting in a waist-high dry bag perched on each bow, secured with surfboard leash hooks and bungee cords. Even when a surprise storm hit the day of launch (the boat captain who dropped us off asked, "Are you sure you want to go, girls? I can take you back to the mainland"), we did fine, paddling through the rain and high surf without much incident.

Sue suggests a walk to a nearby beach; it would be a shame to waste this magnificent forest perched up against the lake. We plunge into the trees, looking for the path that Sue promises is there. Pearl zigzags ahead, driven a little mad, perhaps, by the smells of creatures we can't see. Soon enough, we come upon scat. Sue points and pronounces it bear poop.

"Hold it, there are bears here?" I ask.

My voice is more plaintive than I like. But I am thinking of my tentless sleeping arrangement, the fact I didn't bring rope to haul my toothpaste into high branches. The scat trumpets menace (even though, admittedly, it is unremarkable in size). I try to call upon my vague tracking skills, gleaned only from books and movies. Peering at it, I say, hopefully, "It's not steaming."

"They're timid bears," Sue assures me.

It is hard in this moment not to revert to the prey/predator paradigm I've been steeped in since childhood, all those gory vignettes brought on by *Jaws* or *When Animals Attack*, the poems that see the outdoors as "red in tooth and claw," and the scientists who believe that nature is essentially a battleground. Even the trees around me right now are competing against each other, researchers say, vying for sunlight and nutrients. Otherwise they are inert, dutifully inspiring carbon and exhaling oxygen, growing upward as fast and big as possible, their primary intent (I use that word loosely, because heaven forbid that trees have *intent*) to crowd out others. Yet one only has to slowly walk through a forest, open to its magic, humble in the face of preconceptions, to wonder if trees really are so rapacious. The ecologist Suzanne Simard, for instance, challenges this view. During her three decades studying forests she became convinced that a woodland is a social entity, a living *community*. It is a lively network of intertwined, interacting beings.

According to Simard, trees communicate with each other through a vast subterranean root and fungal system. A forest is, she says, a neighborhood with relationships and an internet of roots and mycelium through which one tree sends carbon, water, and defense chemicals to other trees. Older trees nurture younger ones; younger ones protect older ones, too. If one tree doesn't do well, it's as if a beloved corner store is closing, and trees chemically jump to attention, pumping insect repellent to their neighbor as beetles descend, diverting moisture, offering sugar, offering carbon. Simard's studies suggest that trees reach out not just to their own offspring, but to friends nearby, too, and also to strangers acres away. This is less the floor of Nasdaq, her data seems to show, and more hippie commune, with trees vying to make sure everyone thrives. They're not tribal, either—the ash helps the cedar helps the Jefferson pine. As Simard insists, "trees talk." Let's be clear, there are others who push back on this view, but at this very moment, Simard's paradigm strikes me as fitting: I can almost feel the ground under my feet humming, and I can't help but wonder at what messages might be zipping back and forth, the tree version of gossip. *Humans! Bah! Be on alert all ye saplings!* Or maybe: *Give them some tree energy, those people look like they need it.*

We don't find the path, but we find the beach, which we stomp around on until I say that we should get back, it's getting late. I'm the type of outdoors person who will radically underestimate, say, the strength of the wind at the start of the long ocean kayak paddle, regretting it midway. I routinely misjudge surf conditions, only to have to claw over a succession of incoming behemoths beyond my skill, not always with success.

But it only took being caught out once on a trail as night fell to always add in extra time to get back to camp before dark. I suggest we find that elusive path and return. I've brought a flashlight, because any walk proximate to sunset needs a flashlight, but Sue hasn't, to my surprise. That's okay, I think. I'm the ash to Sue's pine right now.

We get lost. Well, we get lost-ish. The path materializes, then peters out, revealing that it wasn't the right path to begin with. Sue says we should take a shortcut this-a-way. "Oh, the *shortcut*," I tease. "Those famous last words." Seth doesn't know what that means, so I explain how motorists routinely decide at the last minute to exit a highway for a route they see on the map that might save them some time, only to be trapped in a snowstorm, on an unincorporated road, with no cell reception and no chance of people passing by. This isn't just a horror movie genre, it happens in real life repeatedly, I tell him. Sometimes it becomes a heroic survival story, sometimes one of tragedy and death. "Thus 'famous last words,'" I say, feeling sage and godmotherly.

"Famous last words: Look at that nice pack of wild huskies," says Seth.

"Exactly!" I exclaim proudly.

So, lost-ish. We don't panic—this is the beauty of baking in extra time. Instead we take turns hugging a cedar (when you are with a kid, hugging a tree suddenly isn't hokey). Seth shows us the sugar pine, and now we each smell it, swooning over its maple syrup redolence. As we near what Sue promises is our beach, she suddenly points down. Disturbed soil indicates that the fallen tree branch next to it has been moved. "See that?" she says. "A bear pushed this over to look for ants underneath." Sue has tracking knowledge she has been keeping from me, I realize. Not for her the mere steaming scat. She knows how to read the nuances.

"Um," I say, laughing nervously. "Neato?"

We aren't near the beach after all, and we bushwhack for a little while longer, the light fading. But Sue and Seth don't seem worried. They are guessing at the genus of trees, calling for Pearl to stick closer, arguing about the way home.

Despite the unique circumstances of Sue's life now, there is also much about it that tracks with others at this stage. We may not find ourselves parenting a twelve-year-old, but disruptions and changes of circumstances can loom, ranging from retirement to health changes to the death of a loved one. No wonder anxiety is diagnosed more often than depression or cognitive issues in older adults, affecting up to 20 percent of us. Yet it can be avoided, or at least diluted. In the most comprehensive research to date, a Swedish study on almost four hundred thousand cross-country skiers showed that they had a significantly lower chance of developing clinical anxiety. Scientists credit the physical fitness routine for this feat, but what about the fact that these skiers were also working out in the great outdoors? After all, Mother Nature is nonjudgmental about our human foibles, and she'll wrap us in darkness not because of who we are but because her sun sets at this time, a minute earlier than yesterday, and if you misjudge that, well, that's your business.

· · ·

We finally find camp just as civil twilight is pinking the sky. The timing is perfect, despite everything. The three of us shuffle around trying to find flat ground on which to throw down our sleeping bags.

"So what do we do about those bears?" I ask.

"Pearl will scare them away," Sue says.

"Pearl is the size of a house cat," I answer, dismayed. Sue shrugs, remarkably sanguine. She alternates between explaining gently that these South Lake Tahoe bears are wallflowers and throwing declarative sentences at Seth: "Brush your teeth!" "Wash your face!" "Bears are shy, Caroline, it'll be fine." I decide to hope that there is a little Sarge left in there and that she has offered a considered answer, though I know it's more likely she is distracted by parental multitasking, thus picking her battles on the fly. I prop my dry bag against a faraway rock anyway, so my foot is not mistaken for an errant jelly bean or a tube of toothpaste. We get into our sleeping bags and Seth reads from his favorite joke book, insisting we guess the punch line. (*What did one vampire say to another? Answer: Is that you coffin?*) The jokes are terrible (*What do you get when you cross a ghost with a firecracker? Answer: Bamboo*), but we find ourselves laughing anyway. Maybe jokes are like camp food, delicious when consumed outside in nature. Finally, Sue declares, Sarge-like, "Time to sleep."

The sky is too cloudy for stars, but my disappointment quickly dissipates due to the huge silence that surrounds us. It is not the silence of an empty room. It is the deep, nurturing silence of still water, huge slabs of towering rocks, thick cloud cover, no wind. It is the silence of thousands of trees, interconnected, breathing.

Even with my smuggled-in pillow, I wake up constantly. But I don't care. Bits and pieces of favored constellations wink through parted clouds. The quarter moon slides across the sky; I open my eyes to see it to the left, open my eyes again a little while later and it rests above the horizon. At other times, there is no moonlight at all, the sky a deep, thick gray. I decide that fitful rest is perfect; lying under this slowly dancing expanse should not be wasted with deep sleep. I even find myself hoping for a bear. What better way to end this beautiful night than with a magnificent wild creature. Sadly, no bear appears, though I listen intently, rewarded instead by a deep quietude, which becomes almost a sound in itself. (Sue reports in the morning that Pearl, who was attached to her wrist by a leash, excitedly leaped toward the tree line multiple times in the night, dragging Sue's arm with her. Bears, she says, were probably lurking nearby.)

Near dawn it starts to rain. I pull my ground cloth over me and fall back to sleep. A slight chance of drizzle had been predicted, but when I wake again it's still raining. It's summer in California, when rain is almost nonexistent, so perhaps even Sarge would not have predicted this. In fact, at this moment this very rain is causing flash floods all down the middle of California, including a pileup of sixty cars washed from a parking lot in Death Valley National Park. Climate change, climate chaos, climate weirding: call it what you will; it is here. Later I marvel at how desperately humans seem to want stability in their lives, but we won't avert the worst danger to that stability the human race has ever known. For now, though, the three of us know nothing about what is going on just southeast of us. Sue says that the rain doesn't look as if it's going to stop, so perhaps we should pack up with our camp items still wet, and head for home.

The water is glassy and there is little wind. The paddle back is easy. We stay in close formation and, despite the rain, everyone is in a good mood. I had wanted to see in real time how nature helped Sue parent, but I am also struck by deeper lessons, ones that both Sue and I needed to learn. As the rain comes down and the invisible bears recede, I think about how I have always lauded the risk-assessment skills outdoor adventure constantly teaches. Wear the life jacket, bring the flashlight, pack the pillow. Paddle on your knees if you have to. In this way outdoor adventure has given me the confidence to control what I can. But the bigger gift may be the flip side of that coin: the way Mother Nature also asks me to cede control. East wind, yep. Flash flooding in summer, yep. Sudden nephew who is also your son. Yep. You see the conditions and you do what you can to paddle anyway.

Simard believes that trees recognize their own kin. Like humans, trees give their family preferential treatment. Aunts, uncles, cousins, seedlings. They nurture them, Simard says, "with bigger mycorrhizal networks. They send them more carbon below ground. They even reduce their own root competition to make elbow room for their kids." Ahead of me, Sue apprises Seth of their schedule for the day—breakfast, then a shower, then theater camp; *remember to take off that wet shirt as soon as we get to the car so you don't stay cold.* Seth huffs something back. Sue laughs. They paddle toward home, and I follow.

13

Make Waves (Together)

*When you begin as old as me you have the freedom to make as
many mistakes as possible.*

—Lena Salmi, sixty-eight, founder of the Very
Old Skateboarders, who started
skateboarding at sixty-one

There is a whoosh of sound, like an oncoming train. The wave has broken and tumbles toward me in a white frenzy. The water is shallow, so I'm crouched awkwardly; I want to emulate the readiness of a skier at the starting gate, but I instead remind myself of someone trying to find a lost contact lens. The plan is to push off the ocean floor at just the right time, then be carried to shore while clinging prone to a small floatable cafeteria tray called a boogie board. As the white water approaches, I quickly recount the tips I've been given and replay what I've gleaned from watching those on all sides of me—point the board to shore, and when you feel the pressure on your thighs/butt/lower back (one of those, but I'm not sure which), push off. Drop belly onto board. Get weight forward. Hold on. Laugh hysterically.

I'm here in the San Diego surf with about twelve women, mostly in their sixties and seventies, one even in her eighties, who meet multiple times a week on this wide sandy beach to boogie board. I'm interested in why they're so passionate, almost evangelical, about an activity I had barely given much thought to, a sport with aspects of frivolity and play I equated only with those under ten years old, not with women who I imagined might have been made somber, possibly even curmudgeonly, by life and age.

I'm here for the Friday morning session (there will be another at noon). We meet on the sand, all of us in wet suits, me clutching a borrowed board with booties that are too big for my feet. The women are welcoming: friendly, energetic, they introduce themselves in turn. It's winter and the water hovers at a frigid fifty-seven degrees, but that doesn't faze anyone around me. The air is unusually cold for this Southern California beach, too, but that doesn't faze anyone, either, nor does the presence of stingrays, which are common and deliver a mighty stab. Ditto on the possibility of a lurking man-in-the-gray-suit, aka the great white shark; nobody so much as shrugs.

The size of the waves does give them pause, however. Not because they're too big, but because they're too *small*. There has been a bit of sighing and murmuring about this, much as a bunch of teenage surfers might lament that it just wasn't *gnarly* enough out there. Unlike their young counterparts, however, these women seem sure that they'll have a good time no matter what. They're mostly worried that in mild conditions like these I won't understand the true exhilaration of their beloved activity. Will I? I am still puzzled about its allure, but it is clear to me that something about boogie boarding exerts a deep and existential pull, otherwise these women wouldn't be out here, much less come regularly multiple times a week.

The group's founder, seventy-five-year-old Fran Dyer, doesn't at first make things any clearer. "Here's the beauty of boogie boarding," she says, and then proceeds to emphasize the sport's banality. It hasn't changed much since it was first conceived, she tells me, when in 1971 its inventor split a piece of packing Styrofoam in two, rounded one side, and took it into the Hawaiian surf. Also, you don't have to be particularly fit. And it's pretty much a cinch to learn. "You just get on [the board] and go," she explains. "Sure, there are some tricks to catching a wave, but the more you're out there, the more you just get a feel."

Fran also tells me that, unlike many outdoor sports, you don't need a lot of money to partake. Boogie boards are sold at Costco, and wet suits—if you even need them—at thrift stores. Perhaps it is this very demeanor—genial, inclusive, a pickleball of the water—that accounts for much of boogie boarding's magic: it has none of the complexities that adults layer onto the world. This simplicity lays bare boogie boarding's best asset: pure kidlike fun. As Fran explains, it's a chance to shout " 'Yay!!!,' " which you wouldn't otherwise. You can yell and scream all you want, because the ocean is louder than you. Also, the telephone doesn't ring, you don't talk about serious things, and no pressure on anyone."

Today's gathering has its roots twenty years back, when Weight Watchers was a thing and Fran and her friend Christa (now eighty-six and still on the waves) were leaving the meeting and asked the rest of the women there if anyone wanted to go boogie boarding. Ten people joined. Over the years, the group slowly added members. They were an offshoot of the bigger Newcomers Club of San Dieguito, which offered everything from book clubs to hiking for women, but over time the boogie boarder segment, following their sport's laid-back style, opened their sessions and welcomed husbands, children, and grandchildren to the surf. They even recently named themselves: The Wave Chasers, picked from a roster of names that included Salty Sirens and Boogie Board Warriors ("I would have a hard time saying 'Warriors' with a straight face," one member said).

Fran is the perfect boogie board leader, setting this tone of inclusivity and acceptance. "Women would watch us from the beach and come up and say, you're having so much fun, I really want to try it, and we'd put them on our email list." During the pandemic the numbers exploded; today Fran's weekly update of water temperature and weather and her call for who is coming to what session, when, is sent out to more than a hundred people. It's not that everyone sticks with it, Fran tells me. But those who love it and come regularly find deeper meaning. Fran explains that as older women face life changes like retirement, illness, the demise of a marriage, the death of a spouse, they begin to look for adventure and novelty, as well as like-minded friends, all of which this humble ocean activity offers. Fran herself is full of vim and vigor. "Twenty years ago, I thought [seventy-five] was ancient, but I don't feel ancient. I'm still willing to try a new adventure. There are a lot of women willing to do that." This is a revelation to me. I have been on this quest preloaded with the belief that older women *don't* want adventures, even as I've been ferreting out examples of women who embrace exhilaration in the outdoors with the enthusiasm of any twenty-five-year-old. And here's a confession: I've never really boogie boarded. I didn't grow up near the ocean. When I did move to California, I went right to learning to surf. I thought the small foam square and the on-your-stomach technique was something you did only if you were a child, and that it was quickly abandoned at adolescence for something more robust. One friend of mine in her sixties goes out into the ocean every week with her boogie board, but I was sure she was the rare exception, and never delved deeper. Now here is a line of older—even, dare I say it, *elderly*—women decked out in sun hats and full-body wet suits and booties, the freezing ocean at their elbows and the cold wind on their faces, each looking vaguely like a Marvel superhero, and scanning the horizon for their next wave.

Loraine Vaught, sixty-two, joined the group two years ago. Partly it was the pandemic and the need to feel less cooped up. Mostly, though, her fifties had been, as they are for many women, a time of difficult change. Physically, she felt more vulnerable, sure, perimenopause and all that, she tells me. But it was also the aging of the body, which hit her abruptly. All of a sudden, her blood pressure was higher than it had been. She was exhausted all the time. She noticed her balance wasn't as great, and she tore her meniscus. "You're sitting down to stretch and you suddenly you realize, hey, it's hard to get up."

She and her husband also became empty nesters, their one son moving out to take on the world himself. She retired from her job. It seemed that she was no longer contributing to the cultural fabric, and she began to feel of little use in the world. What could she offer? "The fifties are so difficult," she tells me with a shake of her head. "You lose a lot of your confidence." The decisive blow was when her sister died at fifty-seven years old. It was heart-rending and an eye-opener. "I told myself, I better get going."

But get going where? How?

I'm unable to probe further because that wave is incoming. It isn't huge, and it will break before it gets to me; most of the women ride the white water of an already-toppled wave instead of the wave face itself, though one member who later introduces herself as Ginny ("as in gin and tonic") Van Meter, age seventy-six, maneuvers outside the break, and I've been watching her catch the sheer side of each wave, skim down it, and shoot past me with the same half smile each time. She surfed as a young woman, she tells me, but gave it up in grad school. I don't have time to ask her more, but I make a mental note that she probably stopped for the usual reasons—marriage, kids, a new job. When I ask later, she runs me through a vastly different list: a skiing accident that put her in a full leg cast for eight weeks ("which didn't stop me from riding my Honda 90 around the beach, believe it or not"), a crash on a toboggan a few years later, and another ski accident, all of which made knee paddling and popping up on a surfboard darn near impossible. (As an aside, she also explains that she's lived in several countries, once spent four nights in a harem in Saudi Arabia, and dumped a rich attorney "for a drug dealer who whisked me off to Portugal.")

The white water hits and I push off. Some unseen power lurches me shoreward. The sudden speed is heart-quickening. Water taps my face—*Look at you, here, at once a ten-year-old and an almost-sixty-year-old.* Surfing has offered me a similar thrill, but it demands much more technical savvy, and that struggle has always been a distraction from the elemental fun that I am experiencing now. I laugh out loud. Moving with me on the same wave are Loraine, to my right, and Patricia Coe, a retired nurse practitioner, age seventy-five, on my left. These conditions are easy for them, but both are smiling widely anyway. Together, we are skimming toward shore, then some mild error exposes me as a fraud—I'm too far back on my board, it turns out. The engine beneath me rumbles and slows. Patricia and Loraine quickly leave me behind, the soles of their booties all I can see in the froth as they continue to the beach. There is no wave action now, and the sudden loss of power means that I tip inelegantly in the water. It is my first wave, and I now understand much of what the women have been saying. For a moment, at least, I was completely focused. I was deep in play, exhilarated by the speed, immersed in nature—*literally* immersed in it.

I make my way back out to wait for the next wave and try again. Patricia, idling in the water next to me, tells me she joined the group during the pandemic as well. She'd participated in outdoor activities with some younger women, but when she saw an article in the local paper about a group of senior women who boogie boarded, she switched over. She felt that women her age would be able to relate more to her current life experience. She'd been diagnosed with cancer a few years before and had undergone five surgeries. "I realized that survival depended on positive energy, distraction, [and] a challenge, both physical and emotional."

Boogie boarding became what she called "an anchor" in her life. She gained upper-body strength and a sense of purpose. That purpose: to be more fully alive, and to help remind everyone else of that, too. Boogie boarding perfectly aligns with that vision, she tells me, because it is about "laughing with others while sharing tips for an hour in the waves."

Loraine says she had no idea what boogie boarding would come to mean to her when she first sat down on the beach and watched a group of older women in the water looking like they were having some pure, simple fun. Loraine disliked swimming (though she had raced in high school), had no special affinity for the ocean, and had never had an outdoor hobby or lifestyle. Yet she thought, Okay, I know I can do that. She was hooked from the first session. "The thrill of it, when you get a really great wave, riding a wave, there's something about it." Loraine thinks hard about what she's trying to say. "You're *in* the ocean . . . you're really concentrating on the waves, and it keeps you in the moment. You're in the moment for a whole hour."

She tells me that she has never had a job that felt uniquely expressive of who she was, or a hobby that she looked forward to. "This is the first time I really loved something." On the bigger days, when the waves are up to eight feet, she explains that it feels as if she's going "at least sixty miles an hour. The best thing you can do is just hold on." Then, just as she was enjoying the deep focus and the pure physicality of the sport, something else sneaked up on her. She found that boogie boarding had produced a sea change in her confidence.

I immediately want to know more. How could sliding on one's stomach in rushing water change one's sense of self? How does a simple act of play offer such foundational growth? Loraine nods to the horizon, as if to say, look at this vast, intimidating ocean, this cold water, the frigid breeze, the lurking sea creatures, *and I am here.* "Now I know I can do things outside of my comfort zone. I can be uncomfortable and be okay," she explains.

She's trying things that she wouldn't have even considered before she started boogie boarding. Recently, she tells me, she planned a trip that involved a long walk down a steep mountainside. "That's not a big deal to most people," she explains shyly. But to her it was pivotal. She's afraid of heights, and precipitous inclines from the edges of trails are definitely included in this. "But I've been challenging myself to do things with heights," she says. "And I thought, If I can boogie board, I can do this." She walked down the steep mountain trail, no problem.

Socially, she has also begun to reimagine herself. She has never loved the small talk of most gatherings; now she says yes to get-togethers and surprises herself by enjoying them. It's as if overturning her expectations of herself in one area allowed herself to explore more possibilities in others. Still, it's important to note that for Loraine there was no direct through line from her realization that her life had to change to this improbable ocean sport. "I'd never had any outdoors life. I was so wrapped up in raising my son and getting through the day-to-day. But I think I always knew something like that was missing." She had to do a lot of internal clearing, as she calls it, of things she hadn't faced, and needed to, in order to move forward. In the fifties, she says, "there's a reckoning in your own brain. Anything you haven't come to terms with comes back and hits you on the head." She emphasizes that her self-reflection is what ultimately allowed her to be open to something new.

Charlotte Grumbel, the oldest member of the group, greets us standing on the beach in an elegant hat and sweater instead of a wet suit, her aide at her side. She is ninety-seven years old, but it would be easy to mistake her for someone twenty years younger, especially as she explains that she is rehabbing a shoulder strain and then energetically boxes with her arms as if to check the progress she is making. It's not just her shoulder that keeps her out of the water, she tells me—she is also waiting for the warmer water. The last time she was in the surf was last summer, her aide wading in with her and helping with the tricky part, which is less the ride itself than transitioning from a prone to a standing position at the end of it. Charlotte has been boogie boarding since the 1970s, but only learned of the Wave Chasers two years ago. Until then, she simply ventured out on her own, or with her children, grandchildren, and great-grandchildren. I ask her what it is like to be an older woman on the waves. Do people treat her any differently? She laughs and explains that, inexplicably, when young boys spot her they always want to race her. Being the oldest out there, then, is much like being the biggest man in the room, who has to face being constantly (and idiotically) challenged to a fight by younger, smaller guys. "What the boys don't seem to understand is once you're on the wave, we are all going to end up on shore at the same time," Charlotte says, laughing. There is none of that competition among her and her peers, she points out. If there's a goal at all, it is just to find the pure joy in it, no matter what the conditions. "My one regret," she tells me, "is that I didn't find this group earlier."

I came here to investigate the physical aspects of boogie boarding—how its simple skill requirements and forgiving nature might be advantageous as we age. But I am beginning to see that boogie boarding's true value may be rooted in much more, beginning with its uniquely pure aspect of play. To be at play, researcher Stuart Brown says, is to embrace "apparent purposelessness." It is participating in an activity with no clear function, just for the immediate pleasure of it, inviting improvisation, triggering happiness, and experiencing a "suspension of a sense of time." Because of its surface frivolity, play is routinely undervalued by adults, Brown adds; it is dismissed as a luxury, a sign of immaturity, something relegated mostly to childhood. But this attitude is a mistake. "Nothing lights up the brain like play," says Brown in his TED talk on the subject. Among other things, it "fires up the cerebellum, puts a lot of impulses into the frontal lobe, which is the executive portion, and helps contextual memory be developed." Play is the medium through which we socialize, learn, vitalize, and generally experience our world, as integral to the health of the human animal, Brown believes, as dreaming and sleep.

There are many types of play—object play, imaginative play, social play, among others. Boogie boarding is those, but it is specifically "rough-and-tumble play." Much like the full-tilt, chaotic, joyous mock fighting of dogs at a park, many of the playful aspects of being on the waves are in the physical sensations—the cold temperatures, the churning water, the sudden surprising speed. Rough-and-tumble play is the most common kind of play in the animal kingdom, Brown points out. (He begins his book *Play: How It Shapes the Brain, Opens the Imagination, and Invigorates the Soul* with an anecdote about a wild polar bear approaching a husky dog; instead of engaging in a bloodbath, the two begin to play.) During rough-and-tumble play, there is a surprising amount of cooperation (when to run slower, for example, so the little dachshund can catch up a little) and trust (your teeth are bared. Will you draw blood?); animals use this kind of play to learn about each other and themselves.

We can shed so much of our overcivilized selves, then, when we boogie board. This can hold appeal for women, who have been girdled so long by society's constant evaluations and keen attention on our sexual attractiveness, our child-rearing, our career-family balance, our general demeanor. It is at a later stage in life, when those aspects have diminished in currency and we have instead been dropped into a grayer area, that boogie boarding can reorient and guide us. And free us. No wonder it has been such a life changer for so many on these San Diego waves this morning. It is a wild, unruly, at once very personal and deeply social expression of play, offering brain-firing, body-engaging, community-building fulfillment.

"The opposite of play is not work," Brown says. "It's depression."

Aging is a lonely business, we are told, yet here at the Newcomers Club, Wave Chaser division, that isn't evident at all; everyone is milling around, ready to go have coffee now that the session is over. Loraine notes that, even more than a whole string of discoveries—that she loves the ocean, that she can actually embrace the cold, that she now comes to the beach three times a week just for the thrill of a wave—she was most completely bowled over by how much the community aspect of boogie boarding came to mean to her. After she began the sport in earnest, she decided to venture into the surf on her own, and it was fine enough, she tells me, but she was struck by how it was missing an extra zing, some increased delight. There is something about going out in the water with like-minded enthusiasts, she explains. "I've looked down the wave and there are ten people on it, and everyone is giving a little scream with big smiles. We are all experiencing the same emotion at the same time. I love *that*."

Many women start pulling away from connection as they age, says Dr. Louann Brizendine in her book *The Upgrade*. We are embarrassed or overwhelmed, she says, by obstacles like hearing loss, mobility issues, or simply our own shifting sense of identity and place in the world. But retreat is exactly the wrong thing to do. Defining loneliness as "having fewer relationships in which you feel heard and understood than you need to maintain a basic sense of wellbeing," Brizendine notes the many studies that show how isolation can be as detrimental as smoking or lack of exercise to our health as we age.

Brizendine's book focuses on our postmenopausal life, which she regards as an upgrade, not a diminishment. She notes that as our hormones change, so too does our perspective on connection. As our estrogen ebbs, we no longer lead with the "extreme empathy" and bonding habits that often crowded out our own needs; this hormonal shift offers a refocusing onto the self. "We can still lead with love and trust, but with constant lower estrogen, our thinking is no longer overwhelmed by big surges of oxytocin. We have the ability to notice when [our] nervous system is tugged by a familiar yet unhealthy nervous system pattern of another [person]." In other words, the extreme mirroring and caretaking circuitry that women are known and celebrated for during the reproductive years is now replaced, because of a changing endocrine system, with a pathway that routes toward a more self-centered (in a good way) outlook. Put simply, it's "me time," as my gyrocopter instructor Britta Penca had so astutely noted when telling me why older women make such good pilots. Me time still means reaching out to others, but now it's on our own terms.

"Do everything you can to stay connected," Brizendine reminds us enthusiastically. "It's not just longevity we are after in the upgrade; it's joy, emotional strength, and sharpness."

All these traits have been on display this morning on this San Diego beach, and I am humbled by how completely I had underestimated the power of a simple outdoor activity like boogie boarding, especially when it is done in community. Now boogie boards are being swept of their sand and booties pulled off, and the talk is already of the next session. Maybe there will be warmer weather, less wind, bigger waves. Or maybe not. The Wave Chasers will be here anyway, in their neoprene, looking like superheroes and kids and grandmothers, all at once.

14

Ride the Uphills and Downhills

People say oh, be careful, and I think, Hey, you can fall
walking down the stairs. At least if I go out, I go out big.

—JUDY OYAMA, AGE FIFTY-EIGHT, SKATEBOARDER

W hen my mother was fifty-four, she visited my twin
in Los Angeles. At the time, my twin was learning
to become a skydiver and had already taken six or so lessons.
My mother saw an opportunity. She had always wanted "to
do something brave," she tells me now. She decided to join
Alexandra in the air.

This was way out of character for my mother. She grew
up in England discouraged by her own mother from anything
that seemed risky. No sports. No physical play. My mother
remembers that there was "a lot of, you know, looking

anxious. She brought me up to be fearful. I was always afraid." Her mother (my granny) constantly communicated in words or looks, *You shouldn't be doing that. Too dangerous. Be careful, be careful, be careful.*

It wasn't until my mother ventured on a ski trip with friends at twenty-one years old that she realized all the fun she had been missing. The trip was social, the outdoors exhilarating. But, she says, "I was never confident. I was so influenced by my mother and what she said to me. All things were scary." She'd had a glimpse, but that was all. For the next twenty years outdoor adventure remained something forbidding. It was the tumultuous 1960s, but my mother was removed from that, too, never straying from the privileges and expectations of white, upper-middle-class motherhood and housewifery.

Yet she had not forgotten that ski trip. She insisted that we, her children, try everything. Sledding, bicycling, swimming, skateboarding. She didn't do this to improve character or prepare us for a life of courage, resilience, and fortitude. She simply wanted us to be less lonely than she had been. "I didn't have much of a social life," she told me recently, which I had not known, and which broke my heart a little to hear. It seemed impossible that my curious, intelligent, and very beautiful (dark-haired, bright-eyed, high-cheekboned) mother had been lonely. "I decided that sports were the things that gave you a social group. So I was going to encourage you to be sporting, and I remember forcing you into these funny little ski boots at age five. You remember them? I can't remember if it was you or Alexandra, but . . . one of you said to me, 'My feet are so cold.' I took off your ski boots and rubbed your feet." She felt bad about the cold, she said, but not bad enough to let us quit.

The skydive school asked my mother whether she wanted to go tandem—the easier way to experience skydiving—or did she want to jump alone? Alone, my mother answered without hesitation. Jumping attached to the burly chest of someone else didn't count as brave, she'd decided, and if she was going to do this, she would do it all the way. It took a day of instruction. Then it was time to don a bright-yellow suit and enter the jump plane, which was stuffed full with the Danish skydiving team. At altitude, my mother watched them whoop and high-five and then tumble out one by one. My twin jumped, too. Then it was my mom's turn. "The plane had no doors, and I was sitting on the floor, and they said, 'Okay, Sarah, it's time now.' I literally couldn't lift my leg, I was so terrified, and of course they thought that was hilarious. I said, 'I can't move,' and so they got my helmet, then they almost lifted me off and took me to the door." She perched at the opening, twelve thousand feet above the earth, gripping the frame. "I kept saying, 'I can't let go, I can't let go.'" She pauses. "I don't know what happened next, but I think they pushed me."

As my mother dropped (was pushed) from the plane, two instructors joined her in the air. They used hand signals to communicate, Mom explains, "and then they were nodding at my altimeter and I said, 'Oh, right,' and I pulled the ripcord. And they just dropped away. It takes the breath out of you, because it pulls you up, and you're up there in the sky . . ."

My mother interrupts herself here, her eyes shining: "It's *amazing*."

I ask her why, why amazing?

"The feeling," she says. "It was the bravest thing I'd ever done. I was so terrified. And it was so extraordinary to be up in the air looking down at the world."

I have a mental image of my mother skydiving. In it she is set against a blue sky. Her arms are up as if she is being arrested, her cheeks are indented in that uneven way of boxers after a punch. Her eyes are wide, and there is a big, astounded smile on her face.

My mother affixed a Perris Skydiving School sticker to her bumper soon after. She said that it made the car easier to find in a parking lot. But we knew that this was not the whole truth. My mother was proud of her recent adventure. She loved the reminder that she had once been a blaze in the sky. *Daredevil at the wheel!* the bumper sticker now trumpeted. Nothing, not even the ghostly whisper of her own disapproving mother, could take away the fact that my mom had been, irrevocably, without doubt, physically *brave*, if only for one day.

While we talk about her skydiving escapade, my mother mentions to me with typical understatement, or maybe just weird timing, or perhaps simply complete denial, that a few weeks later the very same plane crashed and killed the whole Danish skydiving team.

"What??" I exclaim.

That did not take away the wonder of skydiving for her. It only cemented what she already knew. Skydiving *was* dangerous, but she had jumped anyway.

I don't remember how I felt at the time about my mother's unlikely adventure. I can imagine that I was impressed, but probably didn't say so. I do remember the giddy happiness she felt for a while afterward. I ask now, did skydiving have lasting effects? My mother pauses, mulling her answer. She finally says, "I thought, Now I've done a brave thing." She pauses again, and I can see that it isn't just about the awe-inspiring drop from twelve thousand feet in the air. It's the chasm she had to cross to redefine herself. With one simple step (or push) she'd transformed from a fearful person to someone who had "done a brave thing." Her tone becomes dreamy. "It was very wonderful. You're floating there. You're just up there all on your own."

In the ensuing years, my mother never again jumped from a plane. But that one time served as a powerful primer through which my mother filtered information about her own potential, no matter the messages from the outside world or her own mother. She didn't go so far as to call herself courageous. But as the researchers Becca Levy and Ellen Langer would agree from those studies of how an empowered mindset positively affects aging, this new information (she was someone who could *do a brave thing*) laid down a layer of confidence that in turn boomeranged back to the people around her, who were then also more likely to view her differently. That in turn offered a positive scrim through which she could see herself, and so it goes on and on. It is startling to some that a single experience could change one's concept of oneself deeply, yet look closely at the positive perpetual motion machine that it triggers—experienced by so many of the women in this book—and it is easier to understand. Even today my mother recalls skydiving as one of the most pivotal moments in her life, ranking up there with the births of us, her children.

At age forty, my mother had already abruptly changed course in her life. She'd divorced my father, met a much younger man (he was twenty-eight—this elicited mild disapproval from our small rural East Coast town), eventually completed college, and matriculated to graduate school. All this was an admirable feat of self-determination, and it was hard-won. But when my mother was sixty-two, her life changed again. She and the boyfriend of twenty years split. She retired from her job as a social worker. To cope, she moved to a medium-sized town on the West Coast where there were no memories. Instead, it was almost the blankest of blank slates. With the exception of my brother, who lived a good forty minutes away, she knew no one.

There, she joined a biking group.

I draw a long line from my mother's skydiving adventure more than a decade before to this moment when she resolved to begin road cycling with strangers. The same bravery she discovered in the skies was tapped again, this time on the ground. The group called themselves the Rogue Recyclers, and it was a local club made up mostly of sixty-to-eighty-year-olds. The move must have been intimidating for my mother, not least because of the name, though the reference was to the Rogue River that flowed nearby, rather than any rakish behavior. Joining them might be worth it, my mother thought at the time. It could offer a foothold in her new town, allow her a routine, perhaps make her feel less sad. Maybe, just maybe, she'd even enjoy herself. She had no idea it would change her life, and solidify her sense of herself as a strong, capable woman.

At the time I did not give her credit for the huge step she was taking. She was at an age when women put aside physical challenges, and here was my mother, dusting off a bike that she had bought fifteen years before. It had high handlebars and a broad seat. It was heavy. The salesperson from whom she had bought this bike advised her to use mostly the middle gear, probably because he saw an older woman who would never ride any challenging routes; he had no idea this was a future daredevil at the wheel, or that the country roads where she lived were full of hill and dale. She didn't end up cycling a lot, but when she did, she behaved as instructed and stayed faithfully in the middle gear, laboring up inclines until she had to dismount and push.

For her first ride in her new town, my mother remembers, "I didn't know how to take off the front wheel, so when I put the bike in the car it hung out and I had to leave the back open. I remember meeting them at Phoenix Park. They had proper bike shorts with padding and bike shoes and everything. I had on tights and sneakers and that bike hanging out of the back of the car. I did have a helmet, but that's about all." A woman she had been corresponding with about the ride saw her arrive and went to greet her, and some of the nervousness went away.

Soon my mother was a regular, pedaling twice a week on country roads. Looked at one way, this was a surprise: my mother had long defined herself as unsocial. She wasn't great at gatherings. She didn't like small talk. But biking appealed, she says, "because it isn't like a cocktail party, or sitting next to someone at dinner when you have to talk to them. You could be part of it without the pressure of behaving in a certain way. You can bicycle with someone and then you can kind of leave them and go off if you didn't like them." Bike talk, she explains, is all about which way to turn or *let's stop soon for lunch.* There is no bothersome chitchat. The etiquette was also simple: Help if a tire goes flat. Don't go too fast, don't go too slow. These things she could understand and get behind. "I felt at ease there," she tells me now.

After a while a fellow Rogue Recycler noticed my mother laboring up inclines, and he promptly introduced her to a world beyond the middle gear. My mother was amazed. A "granny gear" with which to hill-climb! And a high gear with which to descend! There is a metaphor here, in the way her world began to open and the way it began to feel easier to live in, despite the terrain. "Naturally, I got a new bike—I couldn't use this old lady bike for long," she tells me. She switched to clip-in pedals. From Ian, my twin's husband, she snagged bright bike shirts emblazoned with corporate names; he was, in addition to being a swim instructor, an expert cyclist of both the road and mountain variety, and soon the two of them were speaking the secret language of velophiles together, about stem length and tire tread and carbon fiber frames.

I'm not a cyclist myself. I biked once with my mom during those years. Believe me, there is nothing more disconcerting than being outpedaled on the road by one's own mother, who also decides to trash talk you as she passes, explains later that she uses "Lance Armstrong's breathing techniques," and suggests that you do, too. Something steely, competitive, and supremely confident had been loosed in my mom through biking, and even as I was being shamed, it was wonderful to see.

Something else happened, too. My British mother had never been overly expressive or affectionate. She came from a tradition steeped in understatement and stoicism. As children, our cuts and bruises were never fussed over, our sibling fights were mostly ignored, and misbehavior, while not tolerated, wasn't overdramatized, either. Yet despite this tough outer shell, my mother's people have always had a deep appreciation for nature—for light rains and stone walls, for good dogs, for clearings in woods, for the flight of quail, for sweeping views at the bend in a country road. They tromp through muddy fields with "wellies" on feet and a walking stick in hand, and as buttoned up as they are, they drop the steely exterior just a bit in the face of natural beauty. This trait began to soar in my mother, and while her American-born peers were describing a ride by degree of difficulty or how long it took, she would say over and over how beautiful it was. I don't think it was a coincidence that during these same years she became more demonstrative, pulling me into a hug spontaneously or kissing my cheek and saying "My beautiful girl!" unprompted. Through biking she had learned to exclaim more often, and grow not just muscular legs but muscular emotions, of appreciation and even exuberance.

For almost twenty years, Mom rode scenic local back roads, took weekend trips to explore new terrain, and entered competitions. (At one registration table a volunteer looked her up and down as she approached and presented her with a thirty-five-mile-race form; she gave the man a withering look and sniffed, "I'm here for the hundred-mile race, thank you.") My mother's happiness and confidence soared. She felt good, she looked good, she was getting outside and having adventures. And even more, she had surprised herself by finding a community within which she flourished.

I watched her new life with respect and pride. She modeled the true potential of elderhood, blossoming after forty, after fifty, then again after sixty. What I did not fully understand at the time was just how impactful this was for my own sense of self—that through this skydiving, cycling-enthused mother I was also being given a continual positive prime about aging. Barring a health disaster (which could come at any age, really) and economic setbacks (also possible at any age), I learned that one's advancing years can be a time of growth and revelation. You march boldly toward the setting sun, marveling at the golden hour, then the twilight, becoming happier and more confident with each step.

When my mother turned seventy-eight, she noticed that her balance was deteriorating. She felt noticeably weaker. When she walked her steps were unsteady, when she biked she wobbled on slow turns. Once she had been one of the fastest cyclists in the group, now she was the absolute slowest. It was startling and disheartening, but she hoped it would pass. She had surgery for a tumor, and the operation went well, though it took a while to recover. Still, she fully expected to continue biking: a measly five-hour operation during which a few ribs were yanked open and some of her lung sliced away wasn't going to keep her from her beloved sport. Once back on her bike, however, she rode with a boozy tilt. She fell a few times. And so, she considered her options. Should she buy a road tricycle, solving her balance issues? Why not join the other cycling club in town, which planned easier rides? But her current car couldn't carry the unwieldy tricycle. Easy rides were what she needed, she knew, but they also weren't very fun. Plus, she was worried that she would wobble into other cyclists despite all her precautions. New bike, new car, new physical limitations, new group—in the end it was too much. Perhaps her own mother's admonitions had finally come full circle. It was too dangerous to get on a bike now. My mother stopped cycling altogether. She was seventy-nine years old.

She didn't talk about the grief she felt. She said at one point that she wasn't sad about it; it was just something that fell away, that she'd changed and lost the passion. The cycling group was different by this time, she said. They weren't interested in being friendly, they were just interested in going fast. But I was pretty sure that I could hear it in her voice. She spoke about cycling the way she spoke of a friend who had died (a lot of her friends were dying around this time). First, the shine in her voice when reminiscing. Then, as the current situation crept in, there was the slowing down of sentences, the practical clip of each word. At the collision of past and present, she would stop speaking for a moment. Twenty years of planning a route with friends, fastening on a helmet, Velcro-ing shoes. Twenty years of legs in orbit, of gear changes, of Lance Armstrong breathing. Twenty years of hills up and hills down, through Oregon springs, summers, and falls. Now gone.

Mom said she never had good balance, but it turned out to be more than that: within a year of putting her bicycle away, she was diagnosed with Parkinson's disease. She seemed almost relieved to know that external sources were responsible for her decision to leave the bike behind, and not her own inherent weaknesses.

What took the place of cycling? Mom worked in her garden. She helped to run a weekly shower truck for people who were unhoused. She gathered food from her neighbors for the local food bank. But bicycling had been something altogether different. By taking up biking, something that would have horrified her own mother, perhaps horrified a whole generation of mothers, she had found community and confidence and physical strength. It took sixty years, but at last those warnings of calamity had stopped intruding on my mother's life. She didn't even need a bumper sticker now. She was *brave*. And she felt, finally, that she belonged. She tells me, "Cycling gave me a feeling of being part of a group. And I never had that before."

My mom still finds ways to be outside. She pulls at errant grasses in her garden, keeps a stern eye on her tomatoes, cuts back the lavender. At least once a day she circumambulates her neighborhood or finds a park nearby to walk in. But there's a hitch in her step. She clasps her hands behind her back as she walks, resembling some pensive French philosopher, perhaps wounded in a war. "You'll get better balance if you swing your arms," I say gently as we putter along a trail. She dutifully brings her arms forward, but can't grasp the rhythm, a result of the Parkinson's, I suspect. Soon she is back to the amble of the melancholy philosopher. Despite all this, the walk has its rewards, evident as she remarks at intervals on how beautiful, stunning, really, the trail is.

My mother's story resonates with me because it is one of triumph over conditioning and societal messaging. It is about the ability to redefine oneself at an older age. It is about searching for and finding community. It is about bravery over fear, growth over stagnation, adventure and change over resignation and quiet. It reiterates how a day full of Dr. Ellen Langer's positive primes—such as the hill you bike up success-fully, or the tire you figure out how to change—really matters; it encourages you to be someone braver, stronger, and more capable of awe and happiness than before. And my mother's story also reminds that, yes, aging is about loss. We lose friends, physical abilities, mental acuity. But it can also be about gains—taking full advantage of what we have until we don't have it anymore. Older age in women is no time to start discarding, my mother's story says. It is a time of embracing as much as possible. It's never too late to do that. Until one day, far down the road, it does become too late. "I hate being eighty-four," she says as we get back in the car. The walk we've just taken was so much shorter than it would have been only six months ago. "What I would give to be sixty again."

That sentence is, I realize, why I am writing this book. There is a melancholy tinge to it, of course. Being old is full of hardship, it says. But it also says something else. My mother isn't yearning to be young. She is yearning to be *sixty*. Who thought that this later stage could be such a time of promise! Certainly, that's not the message we receive from the world around us. Our older years are a time to curl up, give up, they say. Yet the women I have talked to beg to differ. Many have insisted unprompted that this time has been the most rewarding yet. So I look at my mother, as I have looked at all the women I've spoken with, and I am reminded to *do it now*, before I can't. Because why not? It is now crystal clear to me that this final stage can and should be magnificent, thrilling, full of growth and learning and human connection. I am also reminded how beautiful aging can be. My mother blossomed at this later stage. She is still out there, walking, even if it is slowly, looking, exclaiming, feeling, living.

15

Do It Now

If there is one thing I want everyone to learn from this, it's that you should never underestimate grandmothers.

—**CLARE GOIRAN,** MARINE BIOLOGIST, WHO RELIES ON FEMALE CITIZEN SCIENTIST SNORKELERS, MANY IN THEIR SEVENTIES, TO TRACK THE ELUSIVE SEA SNAKE.

My friend Sophia calls and says with excitement, "Oh, wow, there is bioluminescence in Tomales Bay. What do you think, should we go?"

Definitely.

We settle on a date a few weeks away with all the requirements: no moon, tides right, fingers crossed on the weather. We will meet before sunset at a tiny, isolated boat dock far from city lights. At dark, we will launch our stand-up paddleboards and hope for the best—the best being those sparkles of light when this tiny algae species reacts to disturbances by glowing, sparking, winking, *conflagrating* in response. Bioluminescence is one of those odd wonders of nature that, despite its firm scientific explanation, still feels like a mystical experience. (Other things in that category: hail as big as golf balls, the Northern Lights, certain cloud formations, hawk flight.)

At the boat launch I watch fourteen-mile-per-hour winds rake the water and pull a hat down over my ears. Sophia shakes her head. We knew it would be breezier than is ideal—wind not only makes stand-up paddling difficult, it also tamps down the visibility of any bioluminescence in the water—but with the optimism of dumb adventurers everywhere, we came anyway. This is one of the many reasons Sophia is the perfect person for this escapade. We have been close friends for almost forty years, back when someone mistook her for me at a college orientation and then introduced us. To this day, people think we are sisters, even though Sophia is blue eyed and light haired to my hazel eyes and brown hair. We can only speculate that we share the same galumphy way of walking, perhaps, or have a similar ectomorph body type, or perhaps share ten past lifetimes. Whatever it is, people can feel our deep connection.

My wife and her husband are not adventurers of the same ilk, and so we end up relying on each other for all the pursuits that beckon close to our homes—a bike in an unexplored park, a stand-up paddle in the San Francisco Bay, a hike on a new trail. Each outing has excitement similar to a trip in a remote international wilderness, but takes only a few hours. There is little gear, less expense, and no fuss. And Sophia also has the one attribute vital to any adventurer, indeed, anyone going through life: she is game. This was evident when I recently tried to teach her how to ride my Onewheel. I made a sloppy mistake that resulted in her twisting her knee, which I agonized about for some time afterward, until she said to me kindly, "Caroline, we're *adventurers*. This is just what happens."

Now we wait in the car and eat popcorn and watch the sun blaze, then drop behind the peninsula across the water. The sky softens, turning orange and pink. The trees on the ridgeline become silhouettes. We spot the thinnest eyelash of a moon hovering on the horizon. It too sinks behind the trees. The sky melts into purple. I marvel how a sunset happens once every day and yet each time, when we bother to look, it amazes.

We check our watches and change into our wet suits in the last light of day. We sit back in the car with the heat blasting and listen to the wind not die down at all. We point out the island directly in front of us and a quarter of a mile away. This is where we have been told the bioluminescence is most likely. We play word games and talk about her almost grown children and watch the stars appear.

"I think the wind is lessening," says Sophia, meaning, I am now antsy in this car and overheating in my wet suit and maybe we should just go out.

"I think you're right," I agree, meaning, Yes, I am overheating and antsy, too.

Then I add, "What's the worst that could happen?" which is something we often say to each other at the beginning of an outdoor escapade. Sophia usually goes immediately to *The worst that can happen is we die*—which is a true statement in the abstract, but rarely true in a reasonable way. "But we might get lost," I say, and Sophia agrees. There is a pause as we take in the black water, the dark mountains. But we have planned for this: the direction of the tide will push us to land and not out the mouth of the bay to the sea, and the unfortunate wind, which we did not plan, is also in our favor. This means that the worst that could happen is we beach to the south and have to walk a long way. The other worst that could happen, we agree, is that we fall in the water. But we are wearing life jackets and we are leashed to our boards, and we are wearing wet suits to avoid hypothermia. So falling in the water, we reason, is also not a big deal. Finally, we could find ourselves unable to get to shore because of some mysterious, dastardly current (this is very unlikely, but we are exploring all worsts judicially). We remind ourselves that eventually the sun will rise and we could flag down a boat, or the wind will die and we will paddle back to shore. Even if this took eight hours, it would not be catastrophic, just uncomfortable. Satisfied, we don our headlamps and exit the car. Neither of us points out that after all this packing and driving and contorting ourselves into wet suits and then paddling and getting wet and cold, there might be no bioluminescence at all. This would be a disappointment. But it's also just part of the adventure; it doesn't qualify, even as a small whiny aside, for our worst-that-could-happen game.

Right away I realize that we are going to be paddling on our knees; it is too dark to negotiate standing when the water is so choppy. (For someone who once rarely paddled on her knees, this is something I seem to be doing a lot of lately.) For a while there is only the sound of the waves slapping against our boards and the dip of our paddles and the whistling of the wind. And we don't see any signs of biolu-minescence. There are no sparks coming off our paddle strokes, nor are there ribbons of light in our wake. Perhaps we aren't in the right spot yet. We strain our eyes to find that island, which had seemed so obvious just a few hours before, but now on this moonless night has completely disappeared. I switch on my headlamp, but it throws out only a gray murk, illuminating nothing. I switch it off. We're some-where in the middle of the bay now. Isn't this where we want to be? We both stop paddling and sit on our boards. I check the water again and see only a dim gray glow when I pull on my paddle. It's not majestic or breathtaking; it looks as if the night will be a dud for bioluminescence, after all.

Are we disappointed? Not really. The adventure has been in braving the pitch dark, on undulating dunes of water. It has been about looking carefully at the stiff wind and proclaiming it safe. It has been about the soft plunk of a paddle and the low oohs and aahs as we look around us, just over an hour away from our city life and yet in the middle of Mother Nature. It has been about sharing an experience with one of my closest friends.

I think back to a text I'd recently received. It is from Diane Espaldon, the intrepid swimmer. I had been meaning to get in touch, though I had no real expectation that she would continue with swimming or would want to try for the deep end of the pool again. But I thought I would ask anyway. Her text beat me to the punch.

The text features a photo of Diane, in the water, with what appears to be snorkeling gear on her head. She's pulling up her mask and grinning. Floating next to her is a young girl, giving the Shaka-bra sign. Underneath, are the words:

Snorkeling in Guam waters in 20 feet of clear ocean
with Lily and the family. I wore a life jacket but I probably could have done without. Thought of you and Ian
with gratitude.

Reader, I teared up immediately. Forget the deep end of
the pool at eight feet. Diane is paddling around *in twenty feet
of her beloved ocean water.* Sure, with a life jacket, but who cares?
She had once been terrified of water on her face, the deep
chasm below. And here she is, having the fun she's dreamed
of for so long.

At the beginning of this quest I wondered why I saw so
few older women on the adventures on which I embarked.
Turns out, there are women there. Not as many as there could
be, but more than most of us suspect. These women have used
apps, internet searches, social groups, and meetups. They have
enthusiastically practiced outdoor adventure since they were
little girls. They have reluctantly followed loved ones into
nature and found their calling. They have said yes to an
acquaintance who asked them to come outside and play. Ultimately, there are many ways to find your way outside, I now
realize, and there are many kinds of relationships with it once
you are there.

My own views on getting older in the outdoors have
shifted over the course of this book. I began with a relatively
positive outlook on aging, thanks to the example of my own
mother, but I had never fully linked fulfillment in these later
years with the outdoors. All the science I encountered on this
quest was new to me, but now I am deeply convinced, from
the studies that prove that a positive outlook on aging is the
most significant indicator of health and longevity to the

research that proves that Mother Nature offers physical and mental health relief. I was repeatedly bowled over by the ways the women I interviewed were able to continue their outdoor journey by tailoring their adventures to fit their changing circumstances. Mostly, though, I had once been someone who picked extreme outdoor sports to engage in, and now I was agog at how a simpler activity like walking or boogie boarding or bird-watching could entice. These endeavors, I saw, were as immersive, beneficial, awe-inspiring, and fun as anything that had once flooded my nervous system with adrenaline.

One more thing: I am not going outside my lane when I say that this quest has shown me that adventuring outside should be prescribed by doctors and funded by health insurance companies. If you are already an adventurer you may not need that structural incentive, because the women here have shown how vital it is to continue—I salute all your future adventures. If you have never before ventured into the outdoors, however, I hope you are now inspired to begin. There is a bicycle, a pair of binoculars, or an SUP with your name on it. Of course, you may not decide to pursue any of these particular excursions, and that is also excellent. Your outdoor adventure is yours, and it awaits. Just type in *Something fun to do here*, perhaps, and begin.

. . .

Sophia and I have one more trick up our wet suit sleeve. I take out swim goggles and put them on, while Sophia steadies my board. "Don't let me tip," I tell her. She assures me she won't. I maneuver to lie flat. It's awkward, but I twist and bend and finally splay on the board, head toward the water. I can hear the gentle *splish* as the board sways. I remember suddenly a swim lesson at five years old, with the instructor telling us to dunk our tiny heads and blow bubbles. Soph says, "I got you," mistaking my pause for hesitation. I shimmy forward a little more. I take a breath and plop my face into the water. I swirl my hands next to my ears. The universe explodes around me. I am inside a mass of shooting stars. There are blazes of light. More hand swirls produce frantic fireflies, Christmas tinsel, Etch A Sketch white lines. I begin to laugh, the water gurgling. Sparks fly from my breath. I swirl more, lightning flashes. I take my head out, water dripping into my neck. I laugh and laugh. Bioluminescence! We just had to find it on its own terms. Above us, the sky prickles with stars and bright planets, its own sort of light show. The Big Dipper is low and huge on the horizon. The Milky Way hurls itself across the expanse above, our very own galaxy gazing back at this fragile earth, and at us, just two almost-sixty-year-old women whooping in the dark, hair wet, taking another turn at dunking our heads into the dazzling water.

ACKNOWLEDGMENTS

A book is never written on its own.

Thank you to those few who believed that this was possible before I did: my Bloomsbury editor, Nancy Miller; my literary agent, Charlotte Sheedy; and the lovely, incomparable Wendy MacNaughton (as always, thanks for you).

Huge gratitude goes out to my trusted first readers, those people who put aside their own lives to give insight on muddled first drafts. Without you, I'd still have my head in my hands: Bonnie Tsui, there every step of the way saying *You got this, CP*; Alexandra Paul, the one I turn to when I just need someone to say it's great and mean it; Liz Weil, off saving the world a word at a time but who stopped for the manuscript anyway; Sophia Raday, soul sister, sheflexxer, and expert on both writing and on adventure; and Elizabeth Bernstein, indispensable, incisive, but also gentle.

Thank you to the whole Bloomsbury team, who worked so hard to put all these words between covers and get them out into the world. Special notice goes out to Harriet LeFavour, Laura Phillips, cover genius Patti Ratchford, and eagle-eyed copy editor Greg Villepique, with many apologies for not knowing how numbers are written out. To the rest of you at Bloomsbury who make the whole place run, thank you.

So many people stepped up in big ways and small, offering connections, words of writing wisdom, and/or adventure expertise: Louise Aronson, Natalie Baszile, Chris Colin,

Dayton Dabbs, Dan Duane, Chris DeRose, Rodes Fishburne, Jim Garfield, Paul Hollingworth, Elaine Lee, James Nestor, the whole Paul clan, Peggy Orenstein, Shelby Stanger, Julie Spiegler, Miriam Klein Stahl, the San Francisco Writers Grotto.

Shout out to editor Elizabeth Hightower Allen, who advised on an early draft, and editor Mark Lotto, who made a later version so much better.

Thank you to intrepid researcher Lydia Sviatoslavsky.

To those who had my back (and heart) this whole time, you know who you are. You texted, you called, you took me surfing, you took me sailing, you took me snowshoeing in Wyoming. Thank you.

There were many women adventurers who may not have made these pages but were instrumental nonetheless. I either did a deep dive on their lives through research or they personally told me their incredible stories with humility and insight, including Marie Antoine, Lisa Beck, Shannon Coughlin, Jackie G., Annika Granholm, Cherie Gruenfeld, Carolyn Hatfield, Debra Hoteling, Blythe Lasley, Meg Lowe, Tiki Mashy, Nalini Nadkarni, Peggy Oki, Judy Oyama, Lael Robertson, Celeste Royer, Beth Rypins, Pamela Slaughter, Regina Spoor, Janet Allen Williams, the Very Old Skateboarders, and many of the boogie boarders from the Wave Chasers. Your experience and words were all invaluable.

NOTES

CHAPTER 2: LOOK FOR INSPIRATION

22 **"scrubbed from the mythical"** Alisha Haridasani Gupta, "The Mental Health Benefits of an Inclusive Outdoor Escape," *New York Times*, July 14, 2022, www.nytimes.com/2022/07/07 /well/mind/ecotherapy-mental-health-diversity.html.

CHAPTER 3: BUOYANCY MATTERS

35 **In 1958, researchers at the National Institutes of Health** National Institute on Aging, www.nia.nih.gov/research/labs /blsa.

36 **"significantly steeper hippocampal volume loss"** Becca Levy, Luigi Ferrucci, "A Culture-Brain Link: Negative Age Stereotypes Predict Alzheimer's Disease Biomarkers," *Psychology and Aging,* 31(1) 82-88, https://psycnet.apa.org/record/2015-54839 -001.

36 **the opposite is also true** Becca R. Levy and Ellen Langer, "Aging Free from Negative Stereotypes: Successful Memory in China and Among the American Deaf," *Journal of Personality and Social Psychology* 66 (July 1994): 989–97.

36 **an empowering view of aging leads to a longer** Becca R. Levy and Martin D. Slade, "Longevity Increased by Positive Self Perceptions of Aging," *Journal of Personality and Social Psychology*, 81 (2002): 261–70, www.apa.org/pubs/journals /releases/psp-832261.pdf.

36 **"30% better memory scores in old age"** Becca R. Levy, A. B. Zonderman, M. D. Slade, L. Ferrucci, "Memory Shaped

by Age Stereotypes Over Time," *The Journals of Gerontology, Series B: Psychological Sciences and Social Science* 67 (July 2012): 432–36, https://pubmed.ncbi.nlm.nih.gov/22056832/.

36   **her book** *Breaking the Age Code* Becca Levy, *Breaking the Age Code, How Your Beliefs About Aging Determine How Long and Well You Live* (New York: William Morrow, 2022).

36   **Levy also looked at the Ohio Longitudinal Study** Robert C. Atchley, "Ohio Longitudinal Study on Aging and Retirement, 1975–1995," *Harvard Dataverse* 1 (1996), https://doi.org/10.7910/DVN/XL2ZTO.

41   **"intense, amorous contact"** Barry Lopez, *Embrace Fearlessly the Burning World* (New York: Penguin Random House, 2022), 13.

47   **the sometimes excruciating** Tara Roberts, "Into the Depths," *National Geographic*, cover story, Mar. 2022.

48   **"there's something extraordinary about Black people saying, I am going to go out and find my own history, and I'm going to shape the stories that are told about it."** Amy Briggs and Tara Roberts, "The Search for History's Lost Slave Ships," *Overheard at National Geographic*, episode 4, 2020, https://www.nationalgeographic.com/podcasts/overheard/article/episode-4-search-history-lost-slave-ships-overheard.

49   **Interested in the way our subconscious beliefs guide us** Ellen J. Langer, *Counter Clockwise: Mindful Health and the Power of Possibility* (New York: Ballantine, 2009).

50   **"sounded like Lourdes"** Bruce Grierson, "What If Age Is Nothing but a Mind-Set?," *New York Times*, Oct. 22, 2014, www.nytimes.com/2014/10/26/magazine/what-if-age-is-nothing-but-a-mind-set.html.

CHAPTER 4: JUST MOVE

59   **seven thousand to eight thousand daily steps** Gretchen Reynolds, "How Much Exercise Do We Need to Live Longer," *New York Times,* Sept. 15, 2021, www.nytimes.com

/2021/09/15/well/move/exercise-daily-steps-recommended .html?referringSource=articleShare.

59   **more than that doesn't significantly improve your longevity** Amanda E. Paluch, Kelley Pettee Gabriel, and Janet E. Fulton, "Steps per Day and All-Cause Mortality in Middle-aged Adults in the Coronary Artery Risk Development in Young Adults Study," *JAMA Network Open* 4 (2021): 2124516, https://jamanet work.com/journals/jamanetworkopen/fullarticle/2783711.

59   **chance of dying young increases 40 percent** Peter Schnohr, James H. O'Keefe, "U-Shaped Association Between Duration of Sports Activities and Mortality: Copenhagen City Heart Study," *Mayo Clinic Proceedings* 96 (December 2021): 3012–20, www.mayoclinicproceedings.org/article/S0025-6196(21)00 475-4/fulltext.

61   **looks at study after study** Florence Williams, *The Nature Fix: Why Nature Makes Us Happier, Healthier, and More Creative* (New York: W.W. Norton, 2017).

67   **an insect infestation of the emerald ash borer** Geoffrey Donovan, Marie Oliver, "Exploring Connections Between Trees and Human Health," US Department of Agriculture, Forest Service, Pacific Northwest Station. 6p. https://www.fs .usda.gov/research/treesearch/45454.

71   **seventy-two studies** Sebastien F. M. Chastin and Marieke De Craemer, "How Does Light-Intensity Physical Activity Associate with Adult Cardiometabolic Health and Mortality? Systematic Review with Meta-Analysis and Observational Studies," *British Journal of Sports Medicine* 53 (2019): 370–76, https://bjsm.bmj.com/content/bjsports/53/6/370.full.pdf.

CHAPTER 6: CULTIVATE AWE

102 **"and on the boundary of fear"** Dacher Keltner and Jonathan Haidt, "Approaching Awe: A Moral, Spiritual, and Aesthetic Emotion," *Cognition and Emotion* 17 (Mar. 2003): 306.

103 **"when in the presence of vast things"** V. E. Sturm and S. Datta, "Big Smile, Small Self: Awe Walks Promote Pro-Social Emotions in Older Adults," *Emotion* 22 (2022): 1044–58, https://psycnet.apa.org/record/2020-69974-001?doi=1.

103 **"we become more curious"** Annie Murphy Paul, *The Extended Mind* (New York: Mariner Books, 2021), 110.

103 **"enlarges and aggrandizes our sense of self"** Ibid.

104 **researchers from the Memory Care** Sturm and Datta, "Big Smile, Small Self."

104 **"with fresh, childlike eyes"** Gretchen Reynolds, "An 'Awe Walk' Might Do Wonders for Your Well-Being," *New York Times*, Sept. 30, 2020, www.nytimes.com/2020/09/30/well/move/an-awe-walk-might-do-wonders-for-your-well-being.html.

105 **"a very simple intervention"** Nicholas Weiler, " 'Awe Walks' Boost Emotional Well-Being," UCSF Newsletter, Sept. 21, 2020.

106 **"a healthy sense of proportion"** Bryan Robinson, "What Are Awe Walks?" *Psychology Today*, Nov. 3, 2020, https://www.psychologytoday.com/intl/blog/the-right-mindset/202011/what-are-awe-walks.

106 **"producing generosity and generally prosocial behavior** Paul K. Piff, Pia Dietze et al, "Awe, The Small Self, and Prosocial Behavior," *Journal of Personality and Social Psychology* 108, no. 6 (2015): 883–99.

106 **towering old-growth trees** Annie Murphy Paul, *The Extended Mind* (New York: Mariner Books, 2021), 111.

107 **telling helpful stories about themselves** Florence Williams, "The Research on How Awe and Openness Can Help Us Bounce Back from Heartbreak," *MBG Health*, Feb. 3, 2022, https://www.mindbodygreen.com/articles/how-awe-and-beauty-can-make-us-more-resilient-to-heartbreak.

109 **refuse to embrace this last stage** Louise Aronson, *Elderhood* (New York: Bloomsbury, 2018), 89–91.

CHAPTER 7: LEARN SOMETHING NEW

117 **Scientists call this sensation "psychological disequilibrium"** Brenda A. Stevens, Lynette Ellerbrock, "Crisis Intervention: An Opportunity to Change," *ERIC Digest,* US Department of Education, 1995, https://www.counseling.org/resources/library/ERIC%20Digests/95-034.pdf.

117 **Psychological disequilibrium, the research says** Reldan S. Nadler and John L. Luckner, *Processing the Adventure Experience* (Dubuque, IA: Kendall Hunt, 1991).

123 **a human brain can grow and change** *My Love Affair with the Brain: The Life and Science of Marian Diamond,* directed by Catherine Ryan and Gary Weimberg (2017: Luna Productions), https://www.youtube.com/watch?v=OZZJbKzUTFk.

123 **"some losses with age"** Angela Gutchess, "Plasticity of the Aging Brain: New Directions in Cognitive Neuroscience," *Science* 346 (Oct. 31, 2014): 579–82, https://www.science.org/doi/10.1126/science.1254604.

123 **An enriched older brain** Gene D. Cohen, *The Mature Mind: The Positive Power of the Aging Brain* (New York: Basic Books, 2005).

123 **"novelty, focused attention and challenge"** Joyce Shaffer, "Neuroplasticity and Clinical Practice: Building Brain Power for Health," *Frontiers in Psychology* 7 (2016): 1118, http://europepmc.org/article/PMC/4960264.

124 **6 percent of all pilots are women** "Women Pilot Statistics: Female Representation in Aviation," Pilot Institute, April 6, 2023, https://pilotinstitute.com/women-aviation-statistics/.

CHAPTER 8: EMBRACE DISEQUILIBRIUM

150 **"To swim is to be a part of things"** Bonnie Tsui, *Why We Swim* (Chapel Hill: Algonquin Books, 2020), 296.

151 **"build your life around these triggers"** Steven Kotler, *The Art of the Impossible* (New York: Harper Wave, 2021).

CHAPTER 9: FIND YOUR WAY

158 **The more we orient ourselves** Louisa Dahmani and Veronique Bohbot, "Habitual Use of GPS Negatively Affects Spatial Memory During Self-Guided Navigation," *Scientific Reports* 10 (2020): 6310, www.nature.com/articles/s41598-020 -62877-0.

165 **"At the heart of successful navigation"** M. R. O'Connor, *Wayfinding: The Science and Mystery of How Humans Navigate the World* (New York: St. Martin's Press, 2019), 13.

167 **credits the hippocampus for "mapping and sequencing"** M. R. O'Connor, *Wayfinding: The Science and Mystery of How Humans Navigate the World* (New York: St. Martin's Press, 2019), 9.

167 **MRI scans showed that their posterior hippocampi** Eleanor A. Maguire, Kathering Woolett, "London Taxi Drivers and Bus Drivers: A Structural MRI and Neuropsychological Analysis," *Hippocampus* 16, no.12 (2006): 1091–1101, https://pubmed .ncbi.nlm.nih.gov/17024677/.

167 **older volunteers who navigated** Carolyn Wilke, "Navigating a Virtual World Helped Older Adults' Memory," *Scientific American*, June 1, 2020, www.scientificamerican.com/article /navigating-a-virtual-world-helped-older-adults-memory/.

170 **"thinking with your brain alone"** Gaelle Vallée-Tourangeau, Frederic Vallée-Tourangeau, "Beyond the Brain: Cognitive Processes Improve the More You Use Your Hands," *Medical Daily*, Nov. 10, 2016.

CHAPTER 10: ACCEPT LOSS

181 **wholeheartedly rejects the Kübler-Ross paradigm** Meg Bernhard, "What if There's No Such Thing as Closure?" *New York Times Magazine*, Dec. 15, 2021, www.nytimes.com/2021 /12/15/magazine/grieving-loss-closure.html.

186 **"muster hope"** Pauline Boss, *Ambiguous Loss, Learning to Live with Unresolved Grief* (Cambridge, MA: Harvard University Press, 1999).

CHAPTER 11: JOIN IN

189 **competitive sports help youth** Aspen Institute Project Play, "Youth Sports Facts: Benefits," https://www.aspenprojectplay.org/youth-sports/facts/benefits.

203 **"happy people tend to spend more time with others"** "How We Can Learn to Be Happier, with Dr Laurie Santos," South China Morning Post, uploaded Dec. 20, 2019, 6:31, https://www.youtube.com/watch?v=KJTk0Xc-PTw.

203 **"sense of community belonging"** Kenneth M. Kramer and Hailey Pawsey, "Happiness and Sense of Community Belonging in a World Value Survey," *Current Research in Ecological and Social Psychology* 4 (2023): 100101, https://www.sciencedirect.com/science/article/pii/S266662272300014X.

203 **"cultural apparatus"** David Marchese "Yale's Happiness Professor Says Anxiety Is Destroying Her Students," *New York Times Magazine*, Feb. 18, 2022, https://www.nytimes.com/interactive/2022/02/21/magazine/laurie-santos-interview.html.

CHAPTER 12: BE READY FOR CHANGE

221 **trees communicate** Suzanne Simard, *Finding the Mother Tree: Discovering the Wisdom of the Forest* (New York: Knopf, 2021).

221 **"trees talk"** Suzanne Simard, "How Trees Talk to Each Other," TED Summit, 2016, www.ted.com/talks/suzanne_simard_how_trees_talk_to_each_other.

223 **cross-country skiers** Kristen Rogers, "Skiers Might Be at a Lower Risk for Anxiety," CNN Health, Sept. 15, 2021, https://www.cnn.com/2021/09/15/health/skiing-benefits-anxiety-study-wellness/index.html.

226 **"make elbow room for their kids"** Suzanne Simard, "How Trees Talk to Each Other."

CHAPTER 13: MAKE WAVES (TOGETHER)

237 **"apparent purposelessness"** Larry Maguire, "Dr. Stuart Brown on the 7 Properties of Play," *Human Performance*, Feb. 7, 2022, https://humanperformance.ie/the-properties-of-play/.

237 **"Nothing lights up the brain like play,"** Stuart Brown, "Play Is More than Fun," TED Summit 2009, www.youtube.com /watch?v=HHwXlcHcTHc.

238 **"opposite of play is not work"** Stuart Brown, "Play Is More than Fun."

239 **"having fewer relationships"** Louann Brizendine, *The Upgrade: How the Female Brain Gets Stronger and Better in Midlife and Beyond* (New York: Harmony, 2022), 111.

240 **"Do everything you can to stay connected"** Louann Brizendine, *The Upgrade: How the Female Brain Gets Stronger and Better in Midlife and Beyond* (New York: Harmony, 2022).

A NOTE ON THE AUTHOR

CAROLINE PAUL is the author of the *New York Times* bestseller *The Gutsy Girl: Escapades for Your Life of Epic Adventure* and *Lost Cat: A True Story of Love, Desperation, and GPS Technology.* She is also the author of the memoir *Fighting Fire*; the middle-grade book *You Are Mighty: A Guide to Changing the World*; and the novel *East Wind, Rain.* A longtime member of the Writers Grotto, she lives in San Francisco.